"Knowing better does not automate the process of doing better.
Knowing better creates the opportunity for you to choose better."

~ Eric & Maleka Beal

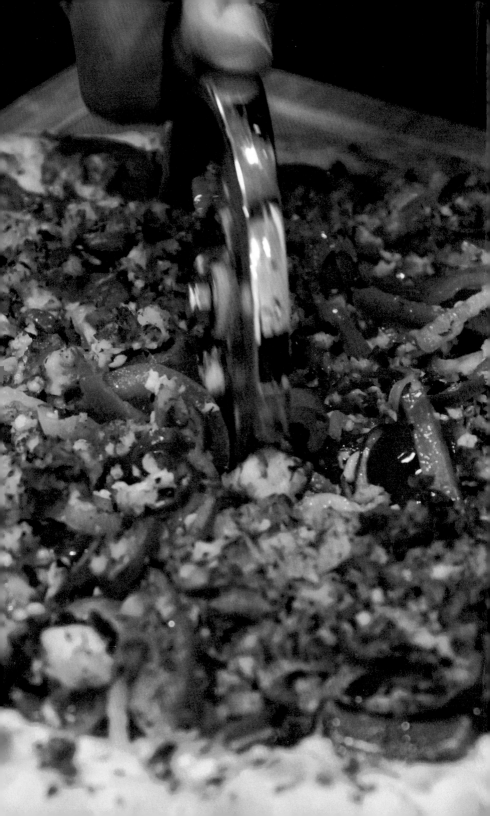

Let's Cook!

BetterChoices Healthy Lifestyle Cookbook

A Guide Inspired by Our Love Affair with Food & Our 300lb Weight Loss Journey

ERIC J. BEAL SR. AND MALEKA J. BEAL

Healthy Lifestyle Coaches & Co-Founders BetterChoices.co

Library of Congress Cataloging-in-Publication Data has been applied for.

ISBN: 0615824536
ISBN-13: 978-0615824536

Visit the BetterChoices website at www.betterchoices.co

Photography by: MJB Design Studio/Maleka J. Beal
©iStockphoto.com/Thomas Perkins, pg 38
Cover & Cookbook Design: MJB Design Studio/Maleka J. Beal

To our sons Eric Jr. and Christopher Beal,
We love you! You are our inspiration.

medical disclaimer

connect with us

for additional programs, books, services, tips, and resources by BetterChoices, please visit us:

- www.betterchoices.co

- www.facebook.com/betterchoicesco

- www.twitter.com/betterchoicesco

- www.youtube.com/betterchoicesco

- www.pinterest.com/betterchoicesco

- www.instagram.com/betterchoicesco

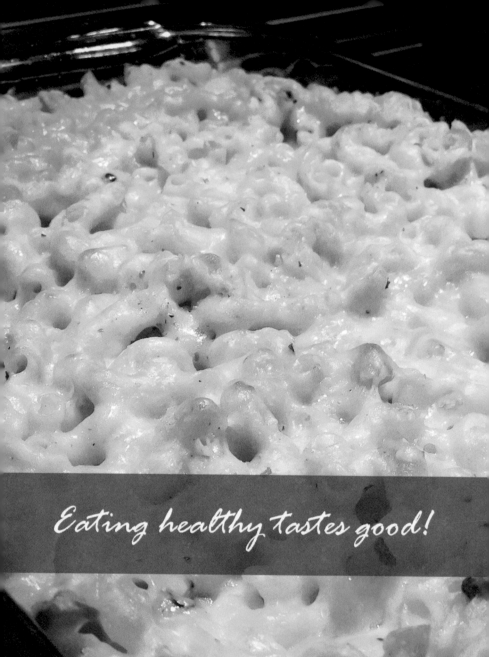

Eating healthy tastes good!

contents

introduction

When we embarked on our weight loss journey 7 years ago, we knew one thing that would NOT change for us -- our love of food and passion for our New Orleans favorites! The truth is, we did not become two very obese individuals by eating wheat grass and drinking vegetable juice...

...WE LOVE TO EAT!!!

Red Beans & rice, fried chicken, po-boys, crawfish etouffee, fish and grits, stuffed peppers, sweet potato pie...these were the foods we grew up on. These were the foods we overindulged in and to be quite frank, we knew we did not want to give these up! We know you can understand because you are thinking of one of your favorites right now!! Here's the deal. We understood, for our journey to be successful, it had to be a LIFEstyle change. This was not about creating a temporary fix; this was about changing our lives. What we didn't know at the time, was how were we going to create this lifestyle change we needed AND incorporate the foods we loved and knew we would not give up. This was the first challenge.

The second challenge was understanding this was a lifestyle change for our family. It's pretty easy to make lifestyle changes for yourself. We were choosing and incorporating changes for everyone -- including extended family and friends. After a lot of research and discussion, we concluded we would need to accomplish three key things for our lifestyle change to be successful and sustainable:

1. We would need to continue to eat the foods we love.
2. We would need to discover healthier ways to prepare them.
3. Preparation and cooking would need to be simple. (...& delicious!!)

As a result, we not only lost a combined 300lbs, we created a framework that transformed every aspect of our thought process and lives. Let us explain...

In 2011, we were thrilled to be participating guests on Oprah's Weight Loss Finale show. After our appearance, we were bombarded with questions! "How did y'all lose the weight?" "What's the secret?" "How long did it take you?" "What did you eat?" "What did you give up?"

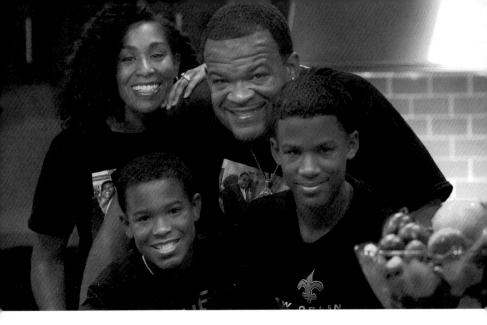

Although each question has a specific answer, the foundation remained the same. We were making BetterChoices.

That same year, BetterChoices was created. Our goal and mission is simple -- to teach, motivate, and empower others to live a healthier LIFEstyle. We wanted to share our knowledge and experience because we knew God did not give us this life experience to keep to ourselves. What we know for sure is the experience of BetterChoices expands way beyond just health...it truly expands to all areas of your life! *(mind, body, and spirit)*

BetterChoices is a healthy lifestyle coaching platform created to teach, motivate, and empower healthy living through empowerment. We want to help you think beyond diet restrictions. We want to encourage you to frame your mind around the idea that you can prepare simple, healthy, and delicious dishes that your family will absolutely love!

Let's Cook! BetterChoices Healthy Lifestyle Cookbook & Guide includes amazing recipes you can prepare for your family, any guests or event! Each dish has the versatility for you to make it your own! It's also a great guide and reference to support you as you create your healthier lifestyle. You will learn about healthier swaps, ingredient equivalents, oils, herbs, and more!

Are you ready to delve in and see what recipes and goodies await you? We hope these recipes inspire you to take control of your health and change the way you view eating--a mindset shift from eating for taste to eating for health and nutrition.

Let's Cook!

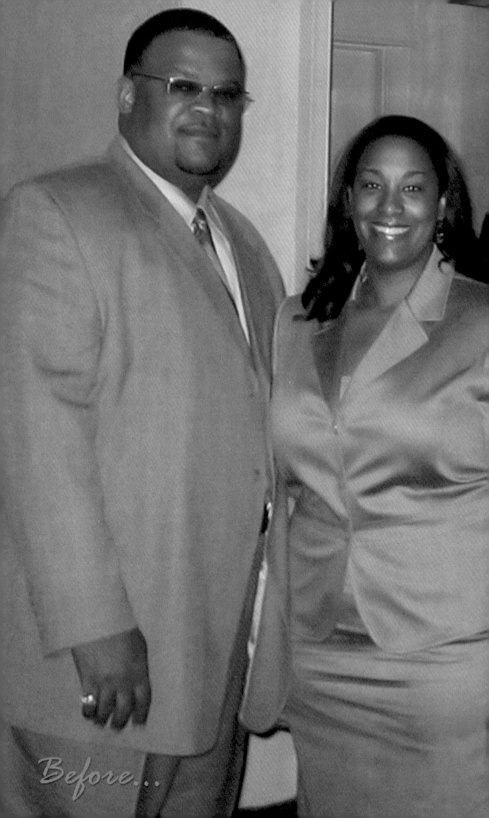

Before...

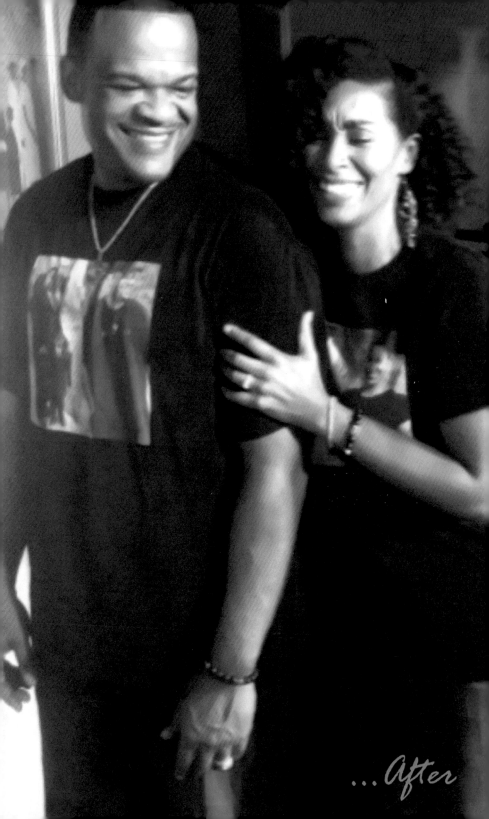

...After

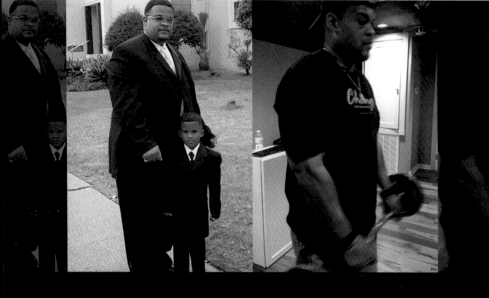

It's a lifestyle.

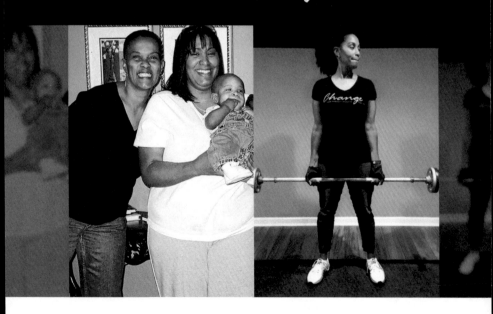

our journey

"When most people are the butt of a joke, they get angry. I got motivated. I had no idea I was 400lbs. Thoughts of dying raced through my mind. I realized, at the time, there are a thousand ways a 35 year old, obese man could die. The only question was, what WOULD I do to change it?"

Did I say obese? …Yep, OBESE! Both of us.

That was my tipping point. Tipping points, by definition, are when small things make a big difference. We go through life asking God questions but many times, we find ourselves unwilling to accept His answers. Even after losing my mother to colon cancer, I still refused to acknowledge the answers that were right in front of my face!

Maleka and I continued going about our everyday lives unwilling to see the bigger picture. That bigger picture was us. (It WAS a really BIG picture!) The bigger picture included our boys, our family, our quality of life, and our future. What kind of future would we have if we continued our bad eating habits, being inactive, and simply, continued not being focused on changing anything about our health and our lives?

Well, we are forever grateful to the nurses who laughed at me. They inspired me to go home, share my experience with my wife, and motivate her to get in this game with me. Just like the movie Bad Boys, "we ride together, we die together," we are committed to this journey and have only looked back to appreciate how far we've come.

At the end of the day, WE ALL KNOW WHAT TO DO. THAT'S NOT ENOUGH! We need to know & understand "how" and "why" what we know will work or not work for us. Understanding things like, "Why can't I eat all foods…fried?" "Why is it not a good idea to eat fast food everyday?" "How can I or why should I get active?" "How or what causes me to gain or lose weight?" "How can I eat the foods that I love AND get healthy?"

Trust us, these are just a FEW questions we asked and answered.

They say a picture is worth a thousand words. Well, for us, our picture is worth AT LEAST 300lbs!!!!

Welcome to BetterChoices! Enjoy the journey!" ~ *Eric & Maleka*

what is betterchoices?

BetterChoices is about change. Change is easy. It's the CHOICE to change that makes us uncomfortable. At BetterChoices, we help you understand **"the how,"** **"the why,"** and **"the what"** you already know, make sense. This is what we call understanding. When you understand something, you can control it. When you can control it, you can conquer it. When you can conquer it, you WIN! It's this understanding that makes the choice to change easier.

Our mission is to teach, motivate, and empower you to change your life by making one betterchoice at a time. Our goal is to help you eliminate the "I don't knows," which are your pre-approved excuses to evade your accountability and responsibility of making the betterchoice.

Our core principles and guiding philosophies:

Tell the Truth! Honesty is the key. It's the foundation required to make your lifestyle change a sustainable success. As stated so eloquently by Shakespeare, "To thine own self be true." You must be loyal to your own best interests.

Know the Options. In any situation or facing any circumstance, the process of resolution has multiple options. So often we rely on what we've been exposed to, never acknowledging that there could be another option, a betterchoice.

It's a LIFEstyle! BetterChoices is NOT a diet. It's not a quick fix. It's a LIFEstyle change. It's about identifying the bad habits you have formed over the years and correcting them one by one. We call these tipping points. Tipping points, by definition, are when small things make a big difference. We help you identify your tipping points. It is your **CHOICE** to change them.

why lifestyle change?

Creating a lifestyle change requires you to take steps and make a self-commitment to change your life. It is a process of changing your mindset or thought process. It's understanding that you are not making a short-term change, you are making a **LIFE**style change.

How we define lifestyle change:
Lifestyle is defined as a way of life or style of living that REFLECTS the attitudes and values of a person or

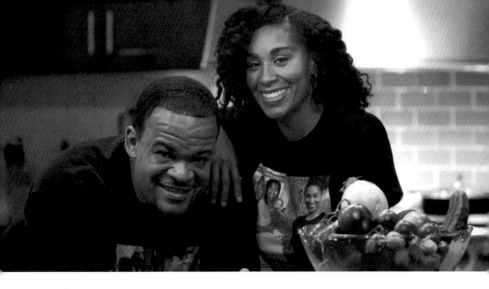

group. Let's break it down into more specific terms:

1. A Way of Life or Style of Living: How do you live now? Are you living the best you can or the best you KNOW how? There is a difference between what we know and what we do. The truth is, we can only do what we know. In order to do something different, we have to LEARN and IMPLEMENT something different.

2. Reflects the Attitudes and Values of a Person or Group: Have you thought about what you reflect to others? What you reflect back to yourself? What does your current lifestyle (eating & exercise habits) say about you? What about the group you associate with? Is everybody healthy? Is ANYBODY healthy? Does your inner circle of family and friends reflect the same habits & CHOICES about their health as you?

The people we associate with REFLECT who we are to ourselves.

Truth is, we become what we do on a consistent basis. Those things we do on a consistent basis are our habits which create our lifestyle.

Most times, our habits are so subtle, we don't really pay attention to them. It is not until we decide we want to create new habits, that we realize just how strong we've allowed our hold habits to become.

Is there an antidote to your bad habits? Yes! YOU!

It is through your "ability" to make BetterChoices that you are empowered to *change your thoughts, change your habits, and change your life.*

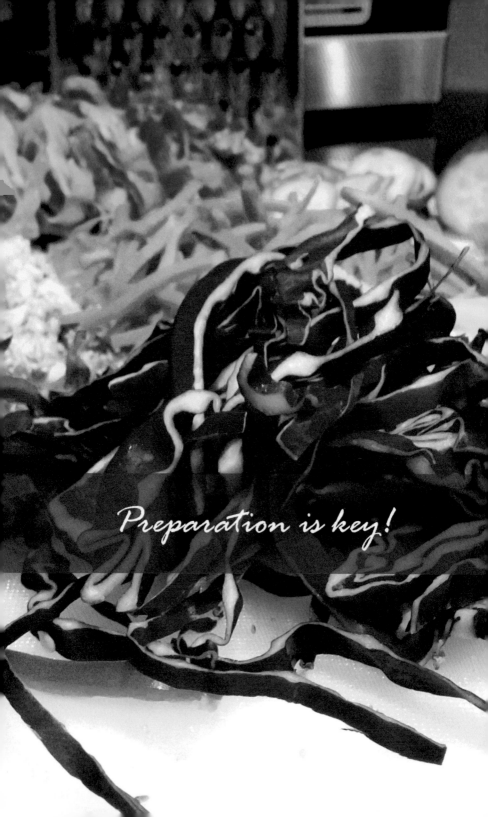

Preparation is key!

Let's get started!

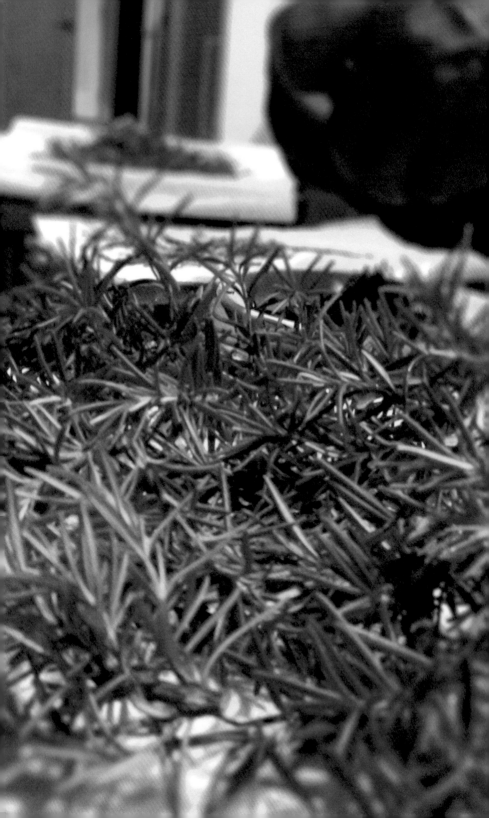

herbs & spices

Every great dish includes delicious herbs and spices! They add a TON of flavor to your foods with minimum calories or other additives. We have compiled a list of robust & flavorful herbs & spices you should keep in your kitchen!

Allspice: Similar to a mix of nutmeg, cinnamon, and cloves. *Add to beef dishes, vegetables, salads, desserts, or just about anything.*

Basil: Member of the mint family. We recommend using fresh basil. *Add to chicken, fish, tomato dishes, pesto, salads and salad dressings.*

Bay Leaf: Mild flavor and are best used dried. Remove before serving. *Add to chicken, seafood, beans, stocks, soups, and pasta sauces.*

Cayenne Pepper: It's all about the heat! This is a very hot spice. Use dried, ground, fresh, and finely chopped. *Add to chicken, seafood, beans, or anything you want to make spicy.*

Celery Seed: Strong celery flavor. Can be added as a replacement to celery. *Add to sauces, soups, vegetables, salads, and salad dressings.*

Chili Powder: Made from red, hot chilies. Heat varies. *Add to bbq sauces, dips, spreads, vegetables, marinades, chili, and mexican dishes.*

Chives: Onion flavor. Recommend use fresh. *Add to potatoes, eggs, salads, sour cream, cream cheese, sauces, and dips.*

Cinnamon: Sweet flavor. Use ground or sticks. *Add to beverages like hot or cold tea, baked desserts, fruits, sauces, meats and chicken.*

Cilantro: Known as Chinese parsley. Used in Latin, Asian, Spanish, and Mexican dishes. *Add to salsa, Mexican dishes, sauces, salads, and salad dressings.*

Cloves: Sweet and savory. Use sparingly. *Add to baked dishes, fruit desserts, sweet potatoes, baked hams, and meat dishes.*

Coriander: Spicy, sweet, & hot. *Add seeds to soups, stews, baked dishes, and vegetables. Add fresh coriander to eggs, cheese, fish, and poultry dishes.*

Dill: Mild and slightly sour. Use as leaves, fresh, seeds, or whole. *Add to fish, eggs, potatoes, meats, salads, sauces, and pickling.*

Fennel Seed: Sweet aniseed flavor. Use ground or whole. *Add to fish, egg dishes, stews, vegetables, salads, salad dressings, and sauces.*

Garlic: Onion flavor. Mildly hot to very hot. Use fresh or granulated. *Add to meats, poultry, fish, Italian dishes, sauces, dips, butters, breads, and marinades.*

Ginger: Peppery flavor. Use dried or freshly grated. *Add to baked dishes, meat, poultry, seafood, and Asian dishes like vegetable stir fry.*

Marjoram: Strong, savory flavor. Use dried or fresh. *Add to fish, poultry, soups, stews, and vegetables.*

Mint: Use dried or fresh. *Add to teas, fruit, poultry, vegetables, and salads.*

Mustard: Simple spice. Use prepared, ground or seed.

Nutmeg: Warm, sweet flavor. Use whole seeds or ground. *Add to baked dishes, sweet potatoes, fruit, vegetables, and sauces.*

Onion: Strong flavor. Sometimes sweet. Use fresh, powder, or dried. *Add to chili, pasta/tomato sauces, meats, poultry, fish, vegetables, and soups.*

Oregano: Similar to Marjoram. Use dried or fresh. *Add to chili, pasta/tomato sauces, vegetables, and soups.*

Paprika: Sweet or Hot. Use dried or ground. *Add to chili, fish, poultry, and potato dishes.*

Parsley: Mild or pungent. Use dried or (we recommend) fresh. *Add to meat, poultry, sauces, eggs, soups, étoufée, beans, and salads.*

Pepper: Vibrant flavor. Varieties include black, white, & green. Use ground or (we recommend) whole black peppercorns and freshly ground it yourself. *Add to just about any dish - eggs, beans, meat, poultry, vegetables, sauces, and more.*

Poppy Seeds: Nutty flavor. Use fresh seeds. *Add to baked dishes, salad dressings, and pasta dishes.*

Rosemary: Very aromatic, piney scent. Use fresh or dried. *Add to meats, poultry, fish, sauces, stuffings, and vegetables.*

Saffron: Very expensive yellow spice. Use as thread or powder form. Use sparingly. *Add to rice dishes, chicken, and fish.*

Sage: Pungent herb. Use fresh or dried. *Add to meat, fish, poultry, stews, stuffings and sausages.*

Savory: Strong flavor. Use dried or whole leaves. *Add to eggs, rice, poultry, vegetables, and soups.*

Sesame Seed: Mild, nutty flavor. *Add to stir fries, poultry, fish, vegetables, salad dressings, and breads.*

Tabasco: Hot spice. Liquid seasoning. *Add to anything.*

Tarragon: Licorice flavor. Use fresh or dried. *Add to eggs, poultry, fish, vegetables, sauces, and salads.*

Thyme: Strong flavor. Use fresh or dried. *Add to meat, poultry, fish, eggs, vegetables, salads, sauces, and stuffings.*

Turmeric: Yellow, pungent flavor. Use sparingly. Dried or ground. *Add to curries and poultry.*

Worcestershire Sauce: Spicy sauce. Liquid seasoning. *Add to meats, ground turkey, sauces, and marinades.*

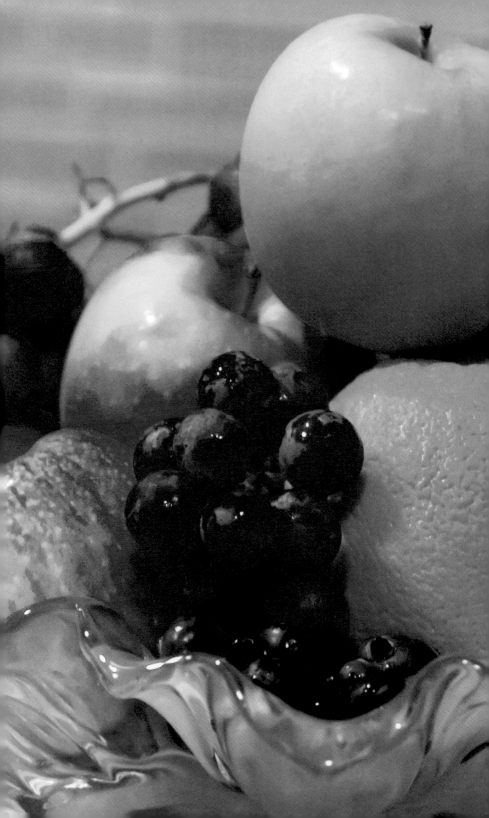

fruit facts

Fruit	Calories	Calories from Fat	Total Fat	Sugar	Protein	Fiber
Apple *1 Large (223g)*	116	3	0g	23g	1g	5g
Apricots *1 cup (155g)*	74	5	1g	14g	2g	3g
Avocado *1 cup (150g)*	240	198	22g	1g	3g	10g
Bananas *1 Medium (118g)*	105	4	0g	14g	1g	3g
Blackberries *1 cup (144g)*	62	6	1g	7g	2g	8g
Blueberries *1 cup (148g)*	84	4	0g	15g	1g	4g
Cantaloupe *1 cup (160g)*	54	3	0g	13g	1g	1g
Cherries *1 cup, pits (138g)*	87	2	0g	18g	1g	3g
Coconut *1 cup, shred (80g)*	283	241	27g	5g	3g	7g
Cranberries *1 cup, chop (110g)*	51	1	0g	4g	0g	5g
Dates *1 date, pit (7.1g)*	20	0	0g	4g	0g	1g
Figs *1 Large (64g)*	47	2	0g	10g	0g	2g
Grapefruit *1/2 Large (166g)*	53	1	0g	12g	1g	2g
Grapes *1 cup (92g)*	62	3	0g	15g	1g	1g
Kiwi *1 Fruit (69g)*	42	3	1g	6g	1g	2g

Fruit	Calories	Calories from Fat	Total Fat	Sugar	Protein	Fiber
Lemons *1 Fruit (58g)*	17	2	0g	1g	3g	2g
Limes *1 Fruit (67g)*	20	1	0g	1g	0g	2g
Mangos *1 cup (165g)*	62	6	1g	23g	1g	3g
Nectarines *1 Large (156g)*	69	4	0g	12g	2g	3g
Oranges *1 Large (184g)*	86	2	0g	17g	2g	4g
Papayas *1 Small (157g)*	68	4	0g	12g	1g	3g
Passion Fruit *1/2 cup (110g)*	97	6	1g	11g	2g	10g
Peaches *1 Large (175g)*	68	4	0g	15g	2g	3g
Pears *1 Large (230g)*	133	2	0g	23g	1g	7g
Pineapple *1 cup (162g)*	82	2	0g	16g	1g	2g
Plums *1 Fruit (66g)*	30	2	0g	7g	0g	1g
Pomegranate *1/2 cup (100g)*	83	11	1g	14g	2g	4g
Raspberries *1 cup (123g)*	64	7	1g	5g	1g	8g
Strawberries *1 cup (166g)*	53	4	0g	8g	1g	3g
Watermelon *1 cup (152g)*	46	2	0g	9g	1g	1g

10 tips to eat more fruit

1. Keep fruits on the counter.
Keep a bowl of fruit on the table, counter, or in the refrigerator IN VIEW. If you see it, you will eat it.

2. Eat fresh, frozen, or dried.
Always try to buy fruits when they are in season. We recommend buying fresh & frozen to ensure you always have fruit on hand. Add to oatmeal, pancakes, protein shakes, or other fruit based recipes. Dried snacks are another great way to enjoy your fruit BUT watch that sugar!

3. Canned fruit is ok.
Be sure when purchasing canned fruits, the fruit is stored in 100% fruit juice or water instead of syrup.

4. Eat fruit for breakfast.
Try adding fruit to your breakfast. Top your cereal or oatmeal with bananas or mix fresh fruit with your low-fat or non-fat greek yogurt.

5. Eat fruit for snack.
Prepare the night before and cut up fruit to add to your lunch. Pack smaller fruit like berries or grapes.

6. Add fruit to salad.
A nice way to enhance any salad is to add fruit. Try adding apple chunks and walnuts or orange slices and almonds to your favorite salad recipe.

7. Eat fruit for dessert
Try baked apples with cinnamon or enjoy cold navel oranges as an after dinner treat.

8. Let kids choose the fruit.
Allow your kids to choose the fruit during your weekly grocery trips. Getting them involved will encourage them to enjoy their healthy choices.

9. Try this Fruit Kabob.
Add pineapples, bananas, grapes, and berries to a kabob stick. Simple, healthy & delicious!

10. Shop Local
Visit your local farmer's market for some new, locally grown fruit you have not tried!

It is recommended you get two (2) servings of fruit every day.

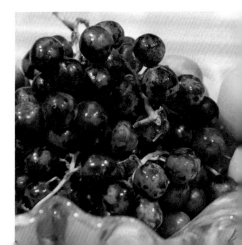

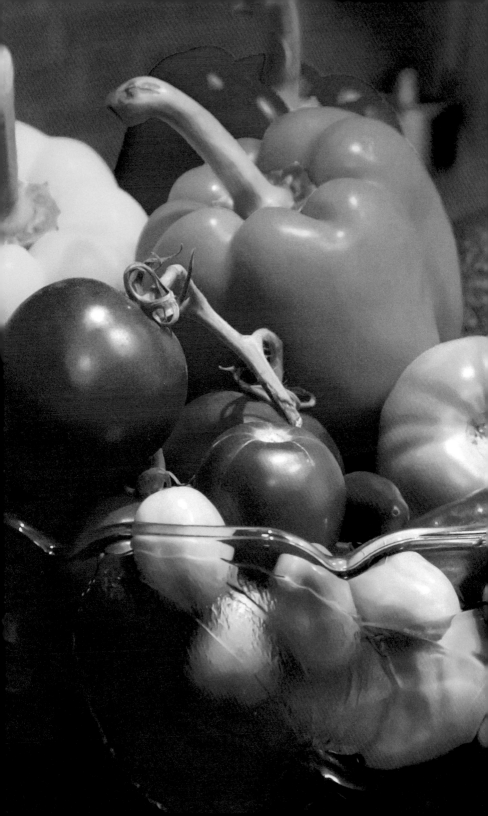

vegetable facts

Vegetable	Calories	Calories from Fat	Total Fat	Sugar	Protein	Fiber
Artichokes 1 Large (162g)	76	2	0g	2g	5g	9g
Arugula 1 cup (10g)	6	1	0g	0g	0g	0g
Asparagus 1 cup (134g)	27	1	0g	3g	3g	3g
Beets 1 cup (136g)	58	2	0g	9g	2g	4g
Bell Peppers 1 Large (164g)	33	3	0g	4g	1g	3g
Black Beans 1 cup (172g)	230	8	1g	4g	14g	15g
Blackeye Peas 1 cup (171g)	200	9	1g	6g	13g	11g
Broccoli 1 cup (91g)	31	3	0g	2g	3g	2g
Brussel Sprouts 1 cup (88g)	38	2	0g	2g	3g	3g
Cabbage 1 cup (128g)	22	1	0g	3g	1g	2g
Carrots 1 cup (128g)	52	3	0g	6g	1g	4g
Cauliflower 1 cup (107g)	27	3	0g	2g	2g	2g
Celery 1 cup (101g)	16	2	0g	2g	1g	2g
Corn 1 cup (145g)	125	18	2g	5g	5g	3g
Cucumber 1 Medium (64g)	47	2	0g	10g	0g	2g

Vegetable	Calories	Calories from Fat	Total Fat	Sugar	Protein	Fiber
Eggplant *1 Large (458g)*	110	8	1g	11g	5g	16g
Fennel *1 Cup (87g)*	27	2	0g	0g	1g	3g
Garbanzo Beans *1 Large (162g)*	270	36	4g	8g	15g	6g
Garlic *1 clove (3g)*	4	0	0g	0g	0g	0g
Great Northern Beans *1 cup (134g)*	27	1	0g	3g	3g	3g
Green Beans *1 cup (83g)*	40	0	0g	3g	1g	3g
Green Leaf Lettuce *1 cup (67g)*	5	0	0g	0g	2g	1g
Iceberg Lettuce *1 cup (57g)*	8	1	0g	0g	1g	1g
Kale *1 cup (67g)*	34	4	0g	0g	2g	1g
Kidney Beans *1 cup (177g)*	230	9	1g	1g	15g	13g
Lima Beans *1 cup (177g)*	220	9	1g	5g	15g	13g
Leeks *1 cup (89g)*	54	2	0g	3g	1g	2g
Lentils *1 cup (177g)*	230	9	1g	4g	18g	16g
Mushrooms *1 cup (70g)*	15	2	0g	1g	2g	1g
Mustard Greens *1 cup (56g)*	15	1	0g	1g	2g	2g
Navy Beans *1 cup (56g)*	15	1	0g	1g	2g	2g

Vegetable	Calories	Calories from Fat	Total Fat	Sugar	Protein	Fiber
Okra *8 pods (95g)*	29	1	0g	1g	2g	3g
Onions *1 cup (160g)*	64	1	0g	7g	2g	3g
Parsnips *1 cup (133g)*	100	4	0g	7g	2g	7g
Peas *1 cup (145g)*	117	5	1g	8g	8g	7g
Pinto Beans *1 cup (213g)*	240	9	1g	1g	16g	14g
Potatoes *1 Medium (213g)*	168	2	0g	1g	5g	3g
Radishes *1 cup (116g)*	19	1	0g	2g	1g	2g
Red Cabbage *1 cup (89g)*	28	1	0g	3g	1g	2g
Red Leaf Lettuce *1 cup (28g)*	4	1	0g	0g	0g	0g
Romaine Lettuce *1 cup (47g)*	8	1	0g	1g	1g	1g
Spinach *1 cup (30g)*	168	2	0g	1g	5g	3g
Squash *1 cup (116g)*	39	1	0g	3g	1g	2g
Turnips *1 cup (130g)*	36	1	0g	5g	1g	2g
Yam *1 cup (150g)*	177	2	0g	1g	2g	6g
Zucchini *1 cup (124g)*	21	4	0g	3g	2g	1g

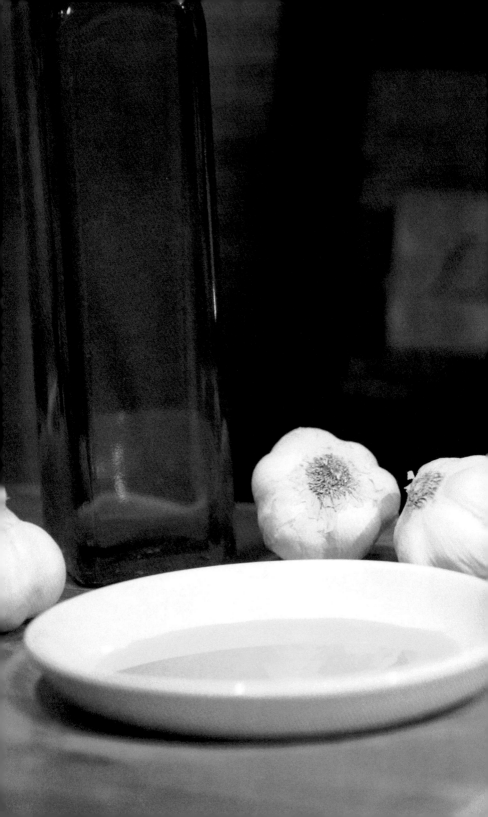

fats & oils 101

All fats are not the same. Certain oils are made for high heat cooking, while others have more intense flavors that are best for drizzling directly on your food.

It's important for you to understand the basics on the various types of oils you will use on your new journey of healthier cooking and eating.

Monounsaturated Fats: These types of fats are tied to cholesterol regulation in the blood, promoting healthy cardiovascular function. Olive, canola, avocado and sunflower are examples of oils with high monounsaturated fat content. *These fats are liquid at room temperature.*

Polyunsaturated Fats: These types of fats include the 'essential' Omega-3 and Omega-6 fatty acids. These play an integral role in several areas—from strengthening our cell structure to reducing the risk of heart attack and stroke. Oils high in Omega-3 fats include flaxseed and fish. *These fats are liquid at room temperature.*

Saturated Fats: There are two main types of saturated fats—animal-based, like lard and plant-based, such as coconut and palm oils. Most of what we consume in the U.S. are artery-clogging, 'long-chain' saturated fats derived from animals.

Plant-based saturated fats are made up of 'short- and medium-chain' fatty acids which our bodies use for energy—this is the reason that oils, like coconut oil, are popular with athletes. *These fats are solid at room temperature.*

Trans Fats: Trans fats are considered unhealthy fats. Like saturated fats, trans fats raise LDL "bad" cholesterol and increase the risk of heart disease. Trans-fats are formed during a chemical process called hydrogenation. This is where cellular chains of fats are artificially altered to create a more solid, stable substance. The result is a fat that is virtually impossible for our bodies to break down.

The take away on trans fats: **AVOID THEM!**

Now that you know the various types of fat, it's important for you to understand the basics of using them when you're cooking.

Whether baking, frying, sautéing, or using oils for dipping, dressing, or marinades, certain oils perform best for each. Let's learn the basics.

types of oils

How do you select the right oil? Great question! We've included a quick list defining a few of the most popular types, as well as, a usage cooking guide.

Avocado Oil: This is a very heart healthy oil. Pressed from avocados, it has a nutty flavor, vibrant green in color, and mild avocado aroma.

Canola Oil: This is a very heart healthy oil due to its fatty acid profile and omega-3 and low saturated fat contents. Good all-purpose oil. Light, golden colored oil perfect for light cooking, sauces and desserts.

Coconut Oil: A heavy, nearly colorless, oil is pressed from the fruit of the coconut palm tree. It is ideal for light and subtly flavored dishes.

Corn Oil: Made from the germ of the corn kernel. It is golden yellow in color. Unrefined oil will have a darker color and richer corn taste.

Grapeseed Oil: It is extracted from the seeds of grapes. This is a by product of the wine-making industry. Light, medium-yellow color. Excellent for salads, raw vegetables, dips, sauces, and salsa.

Olive Oil: Extra virgin olive oil is from the first cold-pressing of olives; mild "pure" olive oil is a blend of refined olive oil and extra virgin olive oil. Olive oil contains heart friendly monounsaturated fat. Oils vary in weight and may be pale yellow to deep green. Excellent for cooking, sautéing, grilling, baking, and stir-frying.

Peanut Oil: Made from pressed, steam-cooked peanuts. It has very subtle scent and flavor. Its relatively high monounsaturated content makes is heart-healthy. Excellent for frying, light sautéing, and stir fries.

Safflower Oil: A golden color with a light texture. Made from the seeds of safflowers.

Sesame Oil: Made from the seed of the sesame plant. It has a high antioxidant content. Comes in two types - a light, very mild, Middle Eastern type and a darker Asian type.

Walnut Oil: Medium-yellow oil with a nutty flavor and aroma.

cooking oil guide

Cooking Method	Fat/Oil (*Unrefined Oils)	Type of Oil	Smoke Point
All Purpose Cooking / High Heat Oils			
Ideal for sautéing, frying, & other high heat cooking. Heat Range: 510°F - 450°F	Avocado Oil	Monounsaturated	510°F
	Safflower Oil	Polyunsaturated	510°F
	Almond Oil	Monounsaturated	495°F
	Soybean Oil	Polyunsaturated	450°F
	Corn Oil	Polyunsaturated	450°F
	Sunflower Oil	Polyunsaturated	450°F
	Peanut Oil	Monounsaturated	450°F
Baking & Sautéing/ Medium High Heat Oils			
Ideal for sautéing, pan-fry, searing, stir-fry, baking, broiling, & grilling Heat Range: 425°F - 350°F	Cottonseed Oil	Polyunsaturated	420°F
	Macadamia Nut Oil	Monounsaturated	410°F
	Sesame Seed Oil	Polyunsaturated	410°F
	Olive Oil	Monounsaturated	410°F
	Grapeseed Oil	Polyunsaturated	400°F
	Canola Oil	Monounsaturated	400°F
	Walnut Oil	Monounsaturated	400°F
	Lard	Saturated	375°F
Light Sautéing & Sauces/ Medium Heat Oils			
Ideal for sauces, baking, salad dressings, low heat grilling, and light sautéing Heat Range: Up to 350°F	Sesame Seed Oil*	Polyunsaturated	350°F
	Coconut Oil*	Polyunsaturated	325°F
	Vegetable Oil	Monounsaturated	320°F
	Olive Oil* (V/EV)	Monounsaturated	320°F
	Peanut Oil*	Polyunsaturated	320°F
	Soybean Oil*	Polyunsaturated	320°F
	Corn Oil*	Monounsaturated	320°F
	Walnut Oil*	Saturated	300°F
	Butter	Polyunsaturated	225°F
	Sunflower Oil*	Polyunsaturated	350°F
	Safflower Oil*	Polyunsaturated	225°F

equivalent guide

US Dry Volume Measurements	
Measure	**Equivalent**
1/16 teaspoon	dash
1/8 teaspoon	a pinch
3 teaspoons	1 tablespoon
1/8 cup	2 tablespoons
1/4 cup	4 tablespoons
1/3 cup	5 tablespoons + 1 teaspoon
1/2 cup	8 tablespoons
3/4 cup	12 tablespoons
1 cup	16 tablespoons
1 pound	16 ounces

US Liquid Volume Measurements	
Measure	**Equivalent**
8 fl. oz.	1 cup
1 pint	2 cups (16 fl oz.)
1 quart	2 pints (4 cups)
1 gallon	4 quarts (16 cups)

Butter / Other Fats	
Measure	**Equivalent**
1 tbsp	1/8 stick
2 tbsp	1/4 stick
4 tbsp (1/4 cup)	1/2 stick
8 tbsp (1/2 cup)	1 stick
16 tbsp (1 cup)	2 sticks
32 tbsp (2 cups)	4 sticks

food equivalent guide

Ingredient	Equivalent Measurement
1 large egg yolk	1 tablespoon + 1 teaspoon
1 large egg white	2 tablespoons + 2 teaspoons
1 large egg	4 tablespoons
1 pound cheese	4 1/2 cups, grated
8-10 large egg whites	1 cup
12-14 large egg yolks	1 cup
3 medium bananas	1 cup mashed
1 egg	1/4 cup egg substitute
3 slices bread	1 cup crumbs
1 lemon	2-4 teaspoons juice 1 tsp grated rind
1 pound tomatoes	1 1/2 cups, chopped
1 pound fresh spinach	12 cups fresh or 1 1/2 cups, cooked
1 pound onions	3 cups, chopped
1 pound cherries	2 1/2 cups, pitted
1 1/2 pounds chicken breasts	3 cups cooked, chopped
1 large onion	1 cup, chopped
1 cup uncooked rice	3 cups cooked white rice
1 cup uncooked pasta	2 2/3 cups cooked pasta
1 pound brown sugar	2 1/4 cups
1 tablespoon fresh herbs	1 teaspoon dried herbs

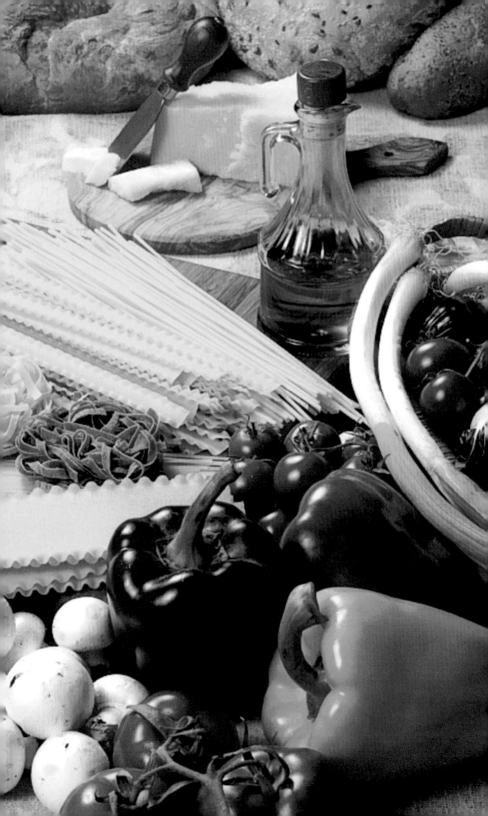

substitution guide

Ingredient Substitutions for Healthier Recipes	
Recipe Ingredient	**Healthier Ingredient Substitute**
Bacon	Canadian bacon, turkey bacon, turkey tasso, or lean prosciutto
Bread, white	Whole-grain/Whole Wheat bread, Pita Bread
Bread crumbs, dry	Panko, Rolled oats or crushed bran cereal
Butter, margarine, shortening, or oil in baked good	Applesauce or prune puree for half of the called-for butter, shortening/oil, or olive oil, unsweetened applesauce, mashed bananas (1 cup mashed bananas = 1 cup oil or butter)
Butter, margarine, or oil to prevent sticking	Cooking spray or nonstick pans
Chicken, dark meat	Chicken, white meat (lower in calories/fat)
Chocolate (M'M)	Dark chocolate (especially in trail mix)
Cookies	Graham crackers or Reduced fat version. Use for pie crusts.
Cream	Fat-Free half and half, evaporated skim milk, coconut milk
Cream Cheese (full fat)	Fat free/low fat cream cheese, Neufchatel, or low fat cottage cheese pureed until smooth
Croutons	Nuts (toasted slivered almonds, pecans, or walnuts)
Eggs	Two (2) egg whites or 1/4 cup egg substitute for each whole egg
French fries	Sweet potato fries
Flour, all purpose (plain)	Whole-wheat flour for half of the called-for all-purpose flour in baked goods, black beans (1 cup flour = 1 cup black bean puree), Nut Flours

Ingredient Substitutions for Healthier Recipes

Recipe Ingredient	Healthier Ingredient Substitute
Frosting	Marshmallow Fluff, Meringue
Fruit canned in heavy syrup	Fruit canned in its own juices or in water or fresh fruit
Ground Beef	Extra-lean or lean ground beef, chicken, or ground turkey
Ice cream	Fruit ice cream (frozen fruit, then puree); frozen yogurt
Lettuce, iceberg	Arugula, chicory, collard greens, dandelion greens, kale, mustard greens, roman, spinach, or watercress.
Mashed Potatoes	Mashed cauliflower, red or sweet potatoes mashed with unsweetened almond milk
Mayonnaise	Reduced-calorie, reduced fat, olive oil based mayonnaise, avocado mash, greek yogurt
Meat as main ingredient	Three times as many vegetables as the meat on pizzas, casseroles, soups, and stews
Milk, whole or evaporated	Reduced-fat or fat-free milk, Almond Milk, Coconut Milk, Soy, Rice Milk / Reduced-fat or fat free evaporated milk
Oatmeal, instant	Steel cut oatmeal, quinoa
Oil-based marinades	Wine, balsamic vinegar, fruit juice or fat-free broth
Pasta, enriched (white)	Whole-wheat pasta, zucchini ribbons, or squash spaghetti
Peanut Butter	Reduced-fat peanut butter or natural peanut butter, almond butter
Potato Chips	Kale chips, sweet potato chips, raw veggies, baked potato slices, popcorn

Ingredient Substitutions for Healthier Recipes	
Recipe Ingredient	Healthier Ingredient Substitute
Rice, white	Brown rice, wild rice, bulgur, quinoa, or pearl barley, grated steamed cauliflower
Salad dressing	Fat-free or reduced-calorie dressing or flavored vinegars
Seasoning salt, such as garlic salt, celery or onion salt	Herb-only seasonings (garlic powder, celery seed, onion flakes) or use finely chopped herbs or garlic, celery or onions
Soups, creamed	Fat-free milk based soups, mashed potato flakes, or pureed carrots, potatoes or tofu for thickening agents
Soups, sauces, dressings, crackers, or canned meat, fish, or vegetables	Low-sodium or reduced sodium versions
Sour cream, full fat	Fat-free or low fat sour cream, plain fat-free or low-fat greek yogurt or cottage cheese
Soy sauce	Sweet and sour sauce, hot mustard sauce, or low sodium soy sauce
Sugar	Reduce the sugar by 1/2; vanilla, nutmeg, or cinnamon or unsweetened applesauce (1:1; for every cup, reduce liquid 1/4 cup, Stevia
Syrup	Pureed fruit or low-calorie, sugar free syrup
Table Salt	Herbs, spices, citrus juices, rice vinegar, salt-free seasoning mixed or herb blends
Tomato Sauce	Sliced tomatoes (on pizza), whole or stewed tomatoes
Tortilla Wraps	Lettuce leaves, Corn tortilla instead of flour tortilla
Yogurt, fruit-flavored	Plain yogurt with fresh fruit slices

10 healthy lifestyle tips

1. This is a LIFEstyle change. BetterChoices is NOT a diet. It's not a quick fix. It's a LIFEstyle change. It's about identifying the bad habits you have formed over the years and correcting them one by one. We call these tipping points. Tipping points, by definition, are when small things make a big difference. As you make small, simple changes, you will yield big results. The key is your consistency & commitment to your lifestyle change.

2. Choose healthier foods. Whether you are grocery shopping, cooking dinner, or eating out, choose healthier ingredients. It is true, you are what you eat. If you feed your body junk, well...that's like putting bad gas in your vehicle. Eventually, your car will begin to run bad, emit bad exhaust, and break down. Your body is the same way. You must choose to treat yourself better! Eat plenty of fresh fruits, vegetables, whole grains, lean meats, low-fat dairy products, and drink plenty of water. It's about providing your body with proper balance. You would be surprised by how many things we experience in our health, skin, hair, etc. are related to or a result of our diet.

3. Eat 5-6 times a day. It's important to keep your body fueled with the right amount of energy throughout the day. When we miss meals, we are actually depriving our body of the proper fuel to function. As a result, you feel tired, unable to focus, and tend to make bad food choices or splurges. Commit to eating 3 meals (breakfast/lunch/dinner) and 2-3 snacks. This will keep your body fueled & help eliminate those cravings.

4. Drink more water. The BEST way to keep your body properly hydrated is to drink water. Water helps to detoxify your body, keep your skin healthy, keeps the bowels regular, aides in digestion, weight loss, and so much more! We discovered in our research that it is best to drink 8oz for every 20lbs of body weight your carry (ex. 150lbs - 7.5 cups or 60oz of water). DRINK UP!

5. Get Active. You MUST get active! Exercise is key to living a healthier lifestyle. It keeps your heart healthy, your body toned, mind sharp, and metabolism revved up! Adding weight lifting to your exercise routine will enhance your body definition and keep your metabolism burning fat and calories even at rest! Try walking after dinner, exercise during commercial breaks, or exercise while you're cooking in the kitchen. The idea is to get in daily activity. Select an exercise routine you love. Why? Because if you enjoy the work, you'll do the work...consistently!

that will change your life.

6. Home = Control. When you prepare and eat meals at home, you maintain control. You are able to prepare your dishes with healthier ingredients. You choose how the foods are prepared, as well as, knowing exact serving sizes and nutritional details. Try preparing some of your restaurant favorites at home. Get the family involved and create new, healthier versions based on your new lifestyle, favorite ingredients, spices, & herbs.

7. Make healthier versions or swaps. Who says you can't have pizza, burgers, or sweet potato pie??!! This is a LIFEstyle not a death sentence! For us, we knew we wanted to continue enjoying some of our favorite foods. We definitely could not think about NEVER having chocolate or pizza, ever again! Whether following one of the recipes in this cookbook or re-creating one of your family favorites, you can make simple, healthier swaps to create new, healthier, & delicious dishes everyone will love!

8. Limit Alcohol. There is no sugar coating this (no pun intended!) Alcoholic beverages offer NO nutritional value to our bodies. It is nothing but sugar and throws a real monkey wrench in your healthy lifestyle & weight loss efforts. As with everything in life, moderation is key. It is important for you to be aware of the empty calories and sugar you consume with each alcoholic beverage.

9. Get a full night of sleep. When God created time, He created 8 hours for rest. Somewhere along the line, we started giving more time to work and less time for self rejuvenation. Sleep is key to your healthier lifestyle and weight loss. A good night's rest will keep you in a great mood, keep you focused and energized for the next day. This is not just for the kids either! You must take your own advice -- Go to bed & commit to getting a full night of sleep, every night. Ok...most nights!

10. Enjoy your life! It is easy to get caught up in the stresses of every day. We think about everything we need to do, everything we forgot to do, everything we think we don't have time to do, blah, blah, blah. Truth is, it's always something. Put things in their proper perspective and make a conscious effort to enjoy your life moments. Stop living your life focused on the things you don't like and spend more time appreciating what you love. Your life is the blessing. Choose life. Choose health. Make BetterChoices.

betterchoices grocery list

Home = Control! Keep your kitchen well-stocked with these healthier foods!

Select whole grains/wheat breads/pastas, low fat dairy, low sodium deli meats & canned items.

lean beef & pork:
- beef tenderloin
- top round
- pork tenderloin
- sirloin
- flank steak
- tenderloin roasts
- filet
- low-fat deli meat
- butterfly pork chops

fresh/frozen seafood:
- sea bass
- halibut
- sole
- flounder
- clam
- salmon
- trout
- cod
- perch
- tuna
- tilapia
- shrimp
- oysters
- anchovies
- sardines
- whitefish
- lobster
- snapper
- swordfish
- catfish
- crab
- crawfish
- scallops
- bass
- mahi mahi

chicken/turkey/poultry:
- chicken
- turkey
- turkey bacon
- low fat deli meat

vegetables:
- asparagus
- broccoli
- cucumbers
- tomatoes
- potatoes
- sweet potatoes
- spinach
- squash
- chilies/perrers
- okra
- greens
- bamboo shoots
- cabbage
- artichokes
- garlic
- lettuce
- beans
- green leafy vegetables
- peas
- corn
- eggplant
- kale
- celery
- seaweed
- bell peppers
- carrots
- onions
- mushrooms
- sprouts

- cauliflower
- grape leaves
- leeks
- bok choy
- rhubarb

fruit:
- apples
- apricots
- bananas
- berries
- grapes
- mangos
- melons
- oranges
- peaches
- nectarines
- tangerines
- pears
- plums
- grapefruit
- lemons
- limes
- plantains
- cherries
- dried fruit
- kiwi
- figs
- olives
- quinces
- currants
- pomegranates

fruit:
- persimmons
- papaya
- zapote
- guava
- starfruit
- litchi nuts
- winter melons
- pineapple
- applesauce

dairy & eggs:
- 1% or skim milk
- almond milk
- soy milk
- rice milk
- greek yogurt*
- cottage cheese*
- eggs
- egg white
- egg substitute
- sour cream*
- unsalted butter
- cream cheese*
- reduced fat cheeses

breads/whole grains:
- bagels
- english muffins
- slice breads
- pita bread
- tortillas
- couscous
- oatmeal
- rice (brown rice, asian rice like jasmine, basmati, or wild rice)
- quinoa
- whole wheat pastas (all varieties)
- bulgur

- cold cereals
- other hot cereals

canned goods:
- tuna (water)
- salmon
- kidney beans*
- garbanzo beans*
- low sodium soups
- canned fruit*
- black beans*
- tomatoes
- tomato sauce/paste
- chickpeas*
- lima beans*
- natural peanut butter

nuts & oils:
- almonds
- walnuts
- sunflower seeds
- mixed nuts
- sesame seeds
- peanuts
- pumpkin seeds
- cashews
- pecans
- olive oil
- peanut oil
- corn oil
- coconut oil
- canola oil
- flaxseed oil
- grapeseed oil
- cooking spray
- sesame oil
- safflower oil

sauces & condiments:
- olive oil mayonnaise*

- salad dressings*
- soy sauce*
- mustard
- ketchup
- hoisin/plum sauce
- hot sauce/tabasco
- honey
- pasta sauces*
- teriyaki sauce*
- vinegars
- taco/chili sauce
- pickles
- jam/jelly
- Worcestershire sauce
- salsa
- steak sauce
- extracts
- broths*
- coconut milk*

herbs:
- basil
- cilantro
- dill/dill seeds
- curry leaves
- garlic
- oregano
- mint
- celery seeds
- peppermint sticks
- rosemary
- thyme
- fennel seeds
- marjoram
- tarragon
- bay leaves

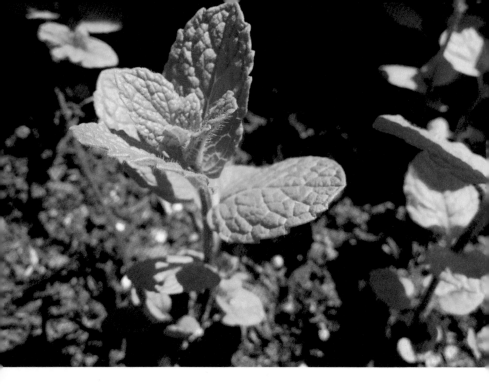

herbs:
- sage
- parsley
- chives
- coriander leaf
- other herbs

seasonings & spices:
- garlic powder
- granulated garlic
- curries
- onion powder
- horseradish
- cumin
- mustard powders
- salt free seasonings
- jalapeño pepper
- cayenne pepper
- black pepper
- red pepper
- lemon pepper
- peppercorns
- salt
- file powder (gumbo)
- pumpkin pie spice
- savory
- all spice
- cardamom
- cinnamon
- paprika
- ginger
- nutmeg
- saffron
- coriander
- caraway seeds
- chili pepper
- clove
- sesame see
- vanilla bean
- other seasonings

baking items:
- flour
- baking powder
- gelatin*
- sugar
- agave
- stevia
- evaporated milk*
- baking soda
- pudding mixes*
- non calorie sweetener
- cocoa powder
- cornstarch

beverages:
- water
- milk (see dairy)
- protein shakes
- protein powder
- vegetable juice*
- coffee
- teas
- crystal light
- carbonated water
- wine (moderation)
- reduced calorie juice
- no calorie mixes

10 grocery shopping tips

1. When shopping for groceries, spend MOST of your time on the perimeter of the grocery store. This is where your freshest ingredients are located. Center aisles are reserved for mostly processed foods. Shop deli, fresh produce, fresh meats, dairy, breads, & frozen vegetables. Lastly, shop the center aisles for things like pastas, cereals, herbs/spices, beans, oils, etc.

2. Look for cereals that have a minimum of 4g or more of fiber, 5g or less of sugar, and 3g or less of fat per serving. Be sure to include hot cereals such as hominy, grits, polenta, etc.

3. There are a variety of dried beans. Consider adding lentils, red kidney beans, navy beans, black beans, black-eyed peas, fava beans, white beans, great northern beans, chickpeas, refried beans, and/or lima beans. Beans are an excellent source of both protein & fiber.

4. The American Heart Association recommends two servings of fish per week. They are a great source of omega-3 fatty acids. In addition, select lean beef, pork, and opt for skinless poultry.

5. When selecting your non-fat/low-fat yogurt, try greek yogurts. They are an excellent source of protein. Be sure to read the labels & be aware of the sugar.

6. When selecting canned foods, be sure to pick items that are low in sodium. Avoid selecting items packed in heavy juices, syrups, or oils.

7. When choosing snacks, select items with whole grains, low sugar, and a very minimal amount of processed foods.

8. When selecting nuts, look for roasted and unsalted.

9. Frozen fruits and vegetables are a great way to keep your home stocked with healthy items. Be sure to add whole grain waffles, bagels, and 100% juices.

10. If the foods you select contains more than five (5) ingredients, artificial, or things you can't pronounce, research it. Probably best not to eat it.

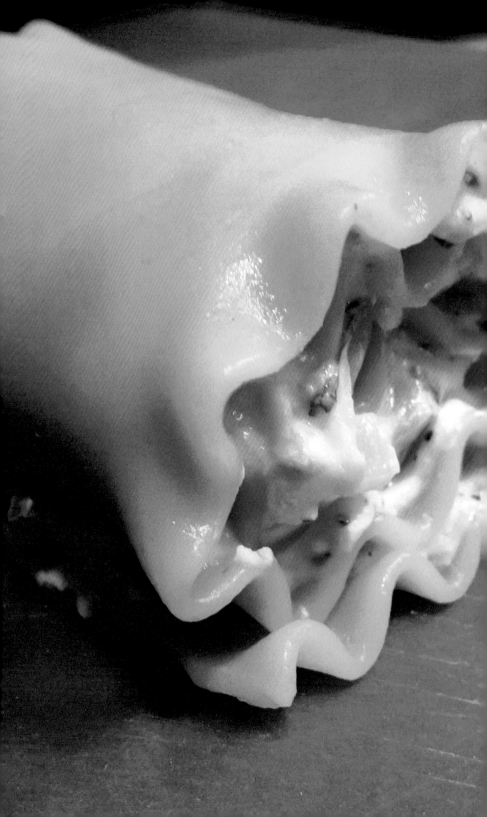

Let's Cook!

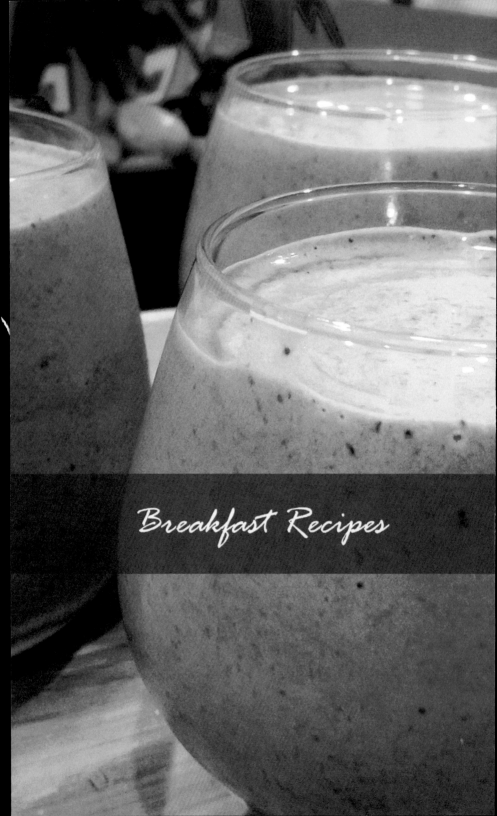

Breakfast Recipes

breakfast tip

Breakfast is the MOST important meal of the day! It fuels your body and your brain so you can be more efficient, focused, and ready to start the day. This is important for your kids too!

Eating a healthy breakfast provides you with numerous health benefits, including weight control and improved performance!

DO NOT SKIP BREAKFAST!

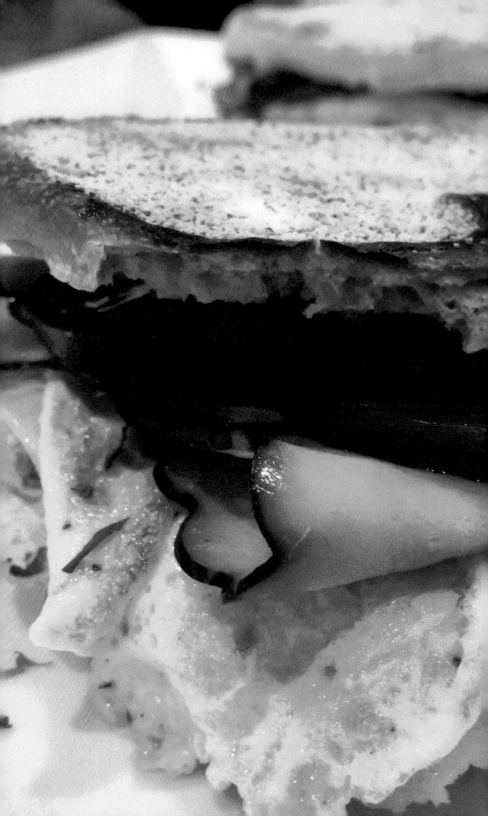

egg & turkey english muffin

Servings: 2

1 large egg
1/2 cup Egg Beaters®
4 oz of sliced turkey (low sodium or home roasted turkey)
1/2 tbsp butter, unsalted
1 tsp parsley
cooking spray
1 tomato, sliced
2 whole wheat english muffins, toasted
sea salt and black pepper

Cut english muffins in half; toast. Set aside. Add eggs and parsley to bowl. Add salt and pepper and whisk eggs until well blended. Spray cooking spray in skillet. Add butter and melt over medium heat. Add eggs and scramble until desired consistency. Remove from heat and set aside. In same skillet, heat turkey until warm. Set aside.

Place english muffins halves on a plate. Divide eggs, turkey, and tomatoes on two halves of the english muffins. Top with remaining muffin halves. Enjoy!

Nutritional Facts: Nutritional information based on one (1) serving or 1 sandwich.
Calories: 262 | **Fat:** 7g | **Fiber:** 8g | **Carbs:** 30g | **Protein:** 27g | **Sugar:** 2g

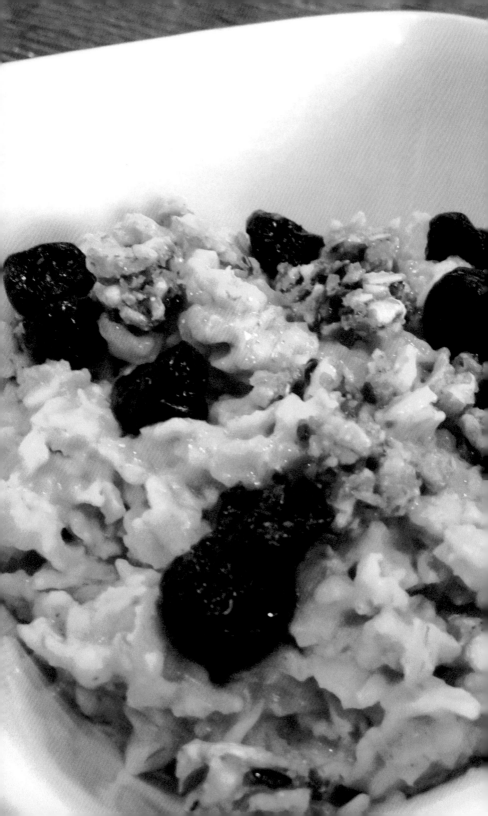

oatmeal crunch

Servings: 2-3

1 cup steel-cut oats
1 3/4 cup vanilla Almond milk, unsweetened
1 tsp cinnamon
1/4 cup Kashi® Go Lean Crunch Cereal
1/2 tbsp unsalted butter
dash sea salt
2 tsp no calorie sweetener, sugar, or brown sugar (optional)
fresh fruit, raisins, or nuts (optional)

Bring almond milk and salt to a light boil in a saucepan. Stir oats into boiling milk. Cook oats until thick and soft, approximately 20 minutes. Stir in butter and cinnamon into cooked oats. Continue cooking for about 5-10 minutes, stirring frequently.

Divide oatmeal into two bowls and sprinkle sugar/sweetener and Kashi® Go Lean Crunch Cereal. Enjoy!

Optional: Swap out Kashi Cereal for fresh fruits/nuts.

Nutritional Facts: Nutritional information based on one (1) serving or 1 cup.
Calories: 225 | **Fat:** 8g | **Fiber:** 7g | **Carbs:** 33g | **Protein:** 7g | **Sugar:** 3g

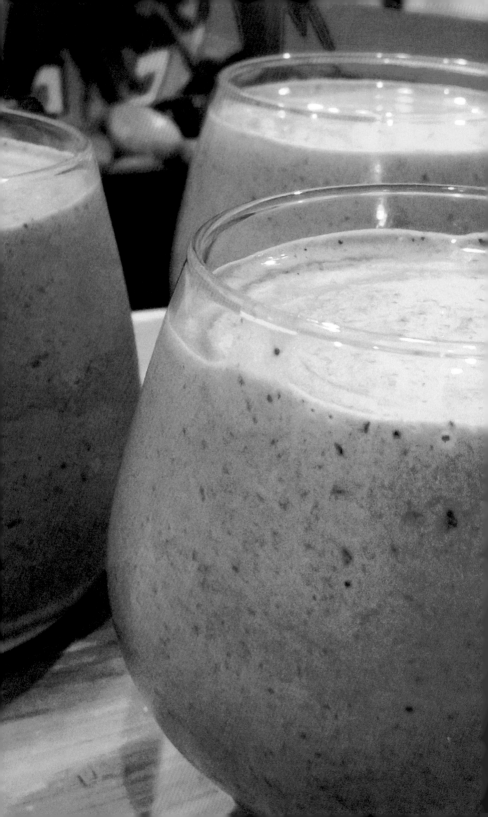

mixed berry protein smoothie

Servings: 2-3

1 cup frozen blueberries
1 cup frozen strawberries
1 1/2 - 2 cups almond milk, unsweetened
2 scoops of protein powder

Combine frozen fruit and milk in blender. Blend until reach desired consistency. May need to add additional almond milk. Add protein powder. Blend well. Enjoy!

Nutritional Facts: Nutritional information based on one (1) serving or 1 cup.
Calories: 170 | **Fat:** 4g | **Fiber:** 4g | **Carbs:** 19g | **Protein:** 14g | **Sugar:** 12g

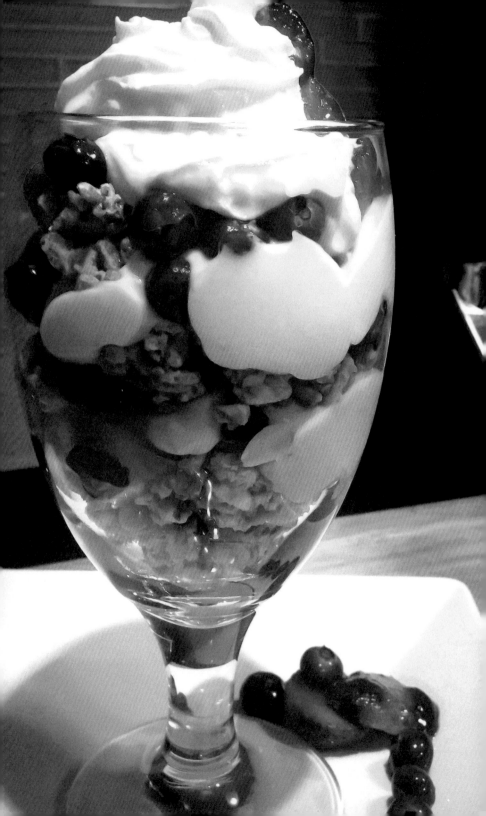

berry almond parfait

Servings: 2

2 5oz nonfat mixed berry flavored Greek Yogurt
1 cup Kashi GoLean® Crunch Honey Almond Flax or Granola
1 cup mixed berries
1 tbsp almond slices (optional)
whipped cream topping (optional)

Layer each parfait glass with 1/4c Kashi, 1/4c mixed berries, 3 tbsp yogurt, 1/4c berries. Repeat layer in each glass. Top with remaining yogurt and almond slices. Enjoy!

Nutritional Facts: Nutritional information based on one (1) serving 1 parfait.
Calories: 258 | **Fat:** 3g | **Fiber:** 8g | **Carbs:** 45g | **Protein:** 15g | **Sugar:** 22g

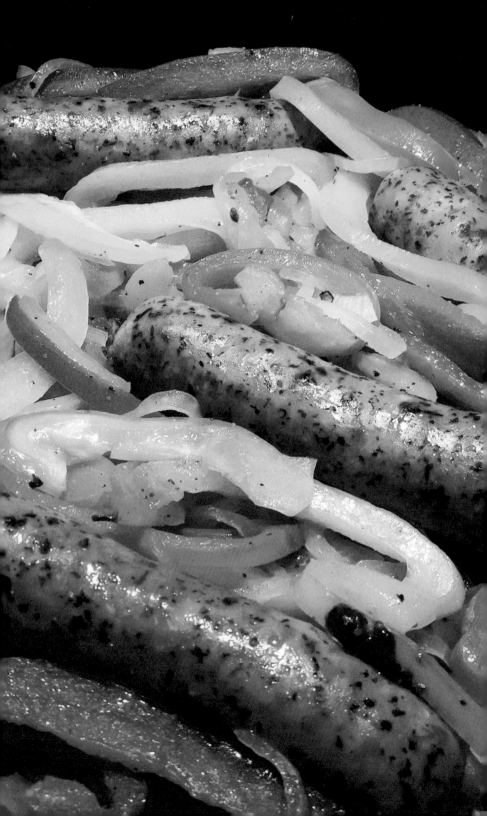

chicken sausage with sweet peppers and eggs

Servings: 5

16 oz (5 links) chicken sausage, sliced
1 tbsp extra virgin olive oil
1/2 green bell pepper, julienne sliced
1/2 sweet red pepper, julienne sliced
1/2 sweet onion, julienne sliced

Scrambled Eggs:
1 large egg
1/2 cup Egg Beaters® Egg Whites
sea salt and black pepper

Spray cooking spray in skillet. Add a little water and place sausage in skillet. Cover skillet. Cook sausage on medium heat, turning often. Cook approximately 10-15 minutes. Remove sausage from skillet and set aside. In same skillet, add olive oil, peppers and onion. Sauté veggies for about 5 minutes. Add sausage and continue sautéing for another 5 minutes. Turn off & set aside.

Spray omelet pan with cooking spray. Set to medium heat. Add eggs to bowl. Season with sea salt & pepper, whisk until well blended. Add eggs to skillet and scramble to preferred consistency. Serve eggs with chicken sausage pepper medley. Enjoy!

Nutritional Facts: Nutritional information based on one (1) serving 1 sausage link.
Calories: 205 | **Fat:** 11g | **Fiber:** 1g | **Carbs:** 11g | **Protein:** 18g | **Sugar:** 7g

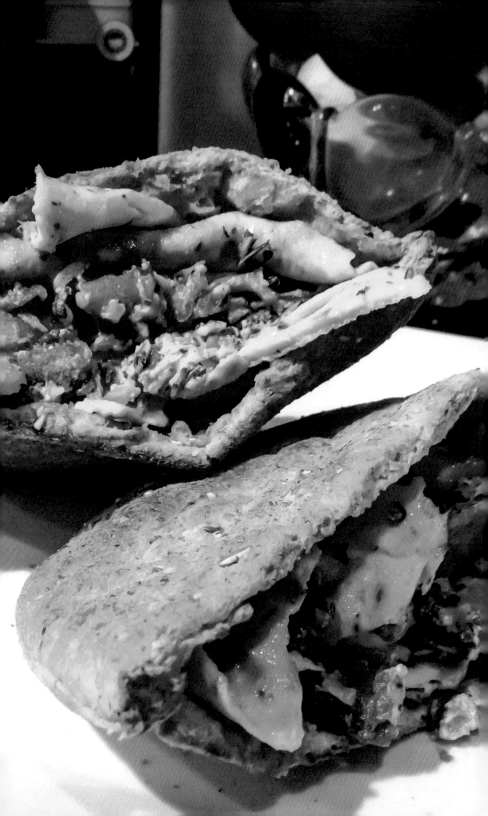

breakfast pita

Servings: 2

1 large egg
1/4 cup Egg Beaters®
4 oz of sliced turkey (low sodium or home roasted turkey)
1 tbsp butter, unsalted
cooking spray
1/2 cup broccoli florets
1 tomato, diced
1 whole wheat pita bread
sea salt and black pepper

Add eggs to bowl. Add salt and pepper and whisk eggs until well blended. Spray cooking spray in skillet. Add butter and melt over medium heat. Add broccoli florets. Saute for about 5 minutes. Add eggs. Scramble until desired consistency. Add tomatoes. Remove from heat and set aside. In same skillet, heat turkey until warm. Set aside.

Cut pita in half. Divide eggs and turkey and fill each pita. Enjoy!

Nutritional Facts: Nutritional information based on one (1) serving or 1 pita.
Calories: 237 | **Fat:** 9g | **Fiber:** 3g | **Carbs:** 14g | **Protein:** 23g | **Sugar:** 2g

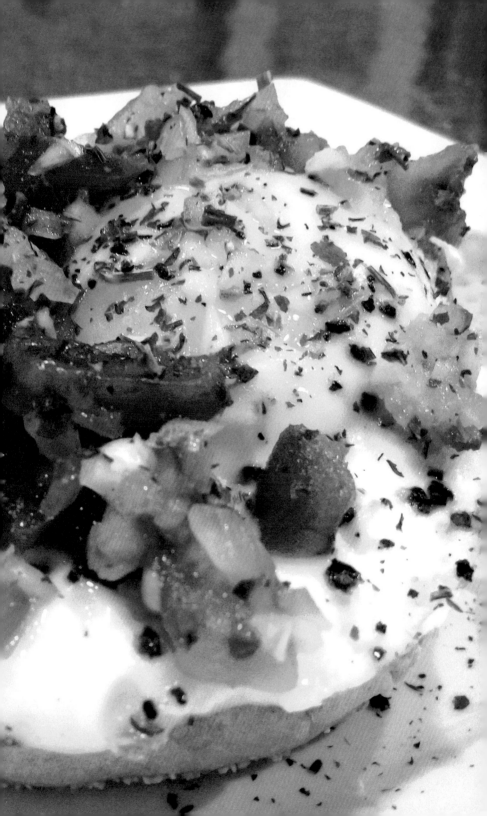

sunny side english muffin

Servings: 2

2 large eggs
4 oz of sliced turkey (low sodium or home roasted turkey)
2 tsp parsley
cooking spray
4 tbsp fresh salsa *(recipe on pg. 151)*
2 whole wheat english muffins, toasted
sea salt and black pepper

Cut english muffins in half; toast. Set aside. Crack eggs in bowl to make sure to avoid any shells & yolk stays in place. Add salt and pepper to eggs. Spray pan and heat over medium-low heat. Gently pour eggs in skillet. Cook over low heat until egg whites are completely set. Cover & continue cooking until yolks begin to thicken but are not hard. Remove from heat and set aside. In small skillet, heat sliced turkey until warm. Set aside.

Place english muffins halves on a plate. Layer muffin with slice turkey, sunny side egg, and salsa. Sprinkle with parsley.

Top with other half of muffin. Enjoy!

Nutritional Facts: Nutritional information based on one (1) serving or 1 muffin sandwich.
Calories: 288 | **Fat:** 7g | **Fiber:** 11g | **Carbs:** 39g | **Protein:** 27g | **Sugar:** 1g

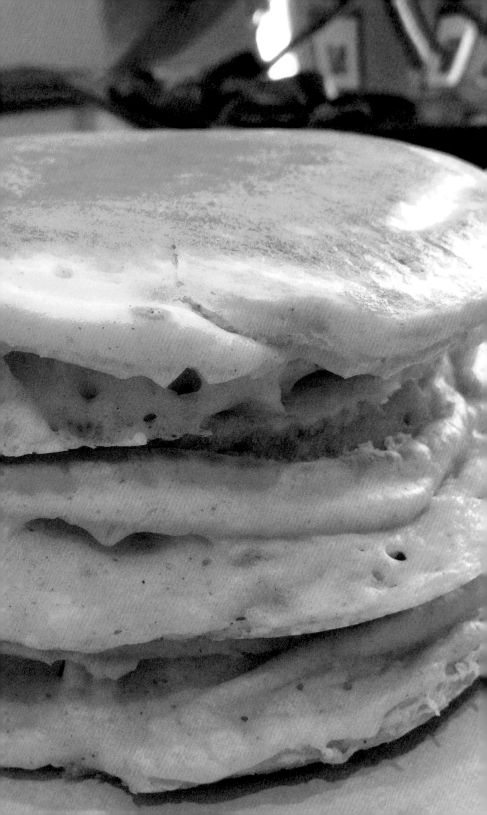

almond pancakes

Servings: 10-12

2 cups Bisquick® original pancake & baking mix
1/2 cup Egg Beaters®
1 cup unsweetened almond milk
2 tsp baking powder
1 tbsp unsalted butter
1 tsp almond extract
1 tsp vanilla extract
1 tbsp no-calorie sweetener of choice

In large mixing bowl, add all ingredients and mix well. Batter will be slightly thick. Add more almond milk to adjust to preferred batter consistency.

Spray large skillet or griddle pan with nonstick cooking spray. Preheat over medium low heat. Pour 1/3 cup of batter onto preheated cooking surface. Cook for 2 minutes per side.

Enjoy with slices of turkey bacon. Top pancakes with favorite fruit.

Nutritional Facts: Nutritional information based on one (1) serving or 1 pancake (1/3 cup).
Calories: 117 | **Fat:** 5g | **Fiber:** 1g | **Carbs:** 16g | **Protein:** 3g | **Sugar:** 1g

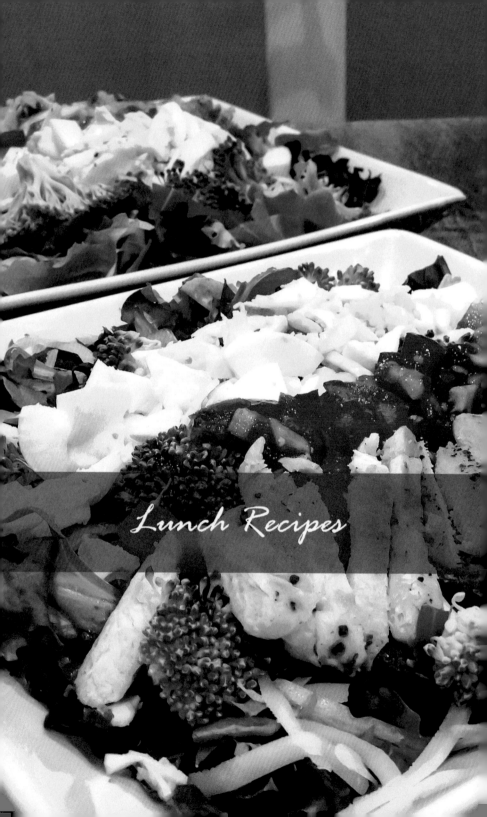

Lunch Recipes

lunch tip

Continue your day, staying fueled, charged, and focused by incorporating healthier lunch choices.

A well-balanced lunch will ensure you have plenty of energy to get you through the day. Stay fueled with lean proteins, whole grains, vegetables, and fruit.

DO NOT SKIP LUNCH!

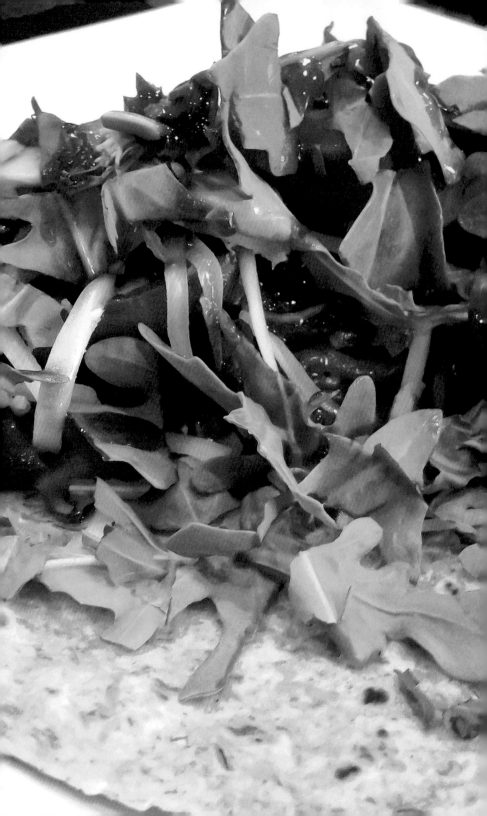

balsamic chicken wrap

Servings: 8

3 boneless/skinless chicken breast, pounded flat
1 onion, thinly sliced
2 tbsp extra virgin olive oil
2 cups arugula, chopped
1 tomato, cubed or Fresh Salsa *(recipe on pg. 151)*
1/4 cup black olives, sliced
1/2 cup light Sour Cream or Non Fat Plain Greek Yogurt
1/2 avocado, sliced
1/2 cup low fat cheddar cheese
Balasamic Vinaigrette
8 Mission® 96% Fat Free Whole Wheat Wraps
sea salt and pepper

Season chicken with salt and pepper. Place chicken breast in large ziploc bag. Pound with meat tenderizer until thin. Heat extra virgin olive oil in a small skillet over medium-high heat. Cook chicken breast until cooked through and juices are clear. Remove from skillet & allow to cool. In same skillet, add onions to skillet & sauté onions until soft and translucent, stirring occasionally. Slice each chicken breast into strips cutting across the breast. Warm Mission® Tortillas.

To Assemble Wraps:
Spread 1 tbsp of light sour cream yogurt in center and expand to edge. Lay 4 chicken strips across middle. Top with cheese, tomatoes/fresh salsa, black olives, grilled onions, avocado slices, and top with arugula. Drizzle 1/2 tsp of balsamic vinaigrette. Enjoy!

Nutritional Facts: Nutritional information based on one (1) serving or 1 wrap.
Calories: 286 | **Fat:** 13g | **Fiber:** 4g | **Carbs:** 27g | **Protein:** 18g | **Sugar:** 4g

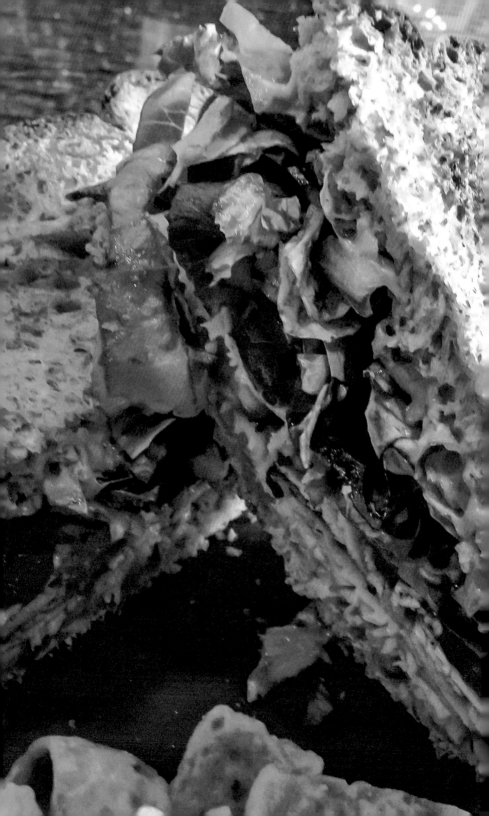

turkey sandwich

Servings: 1

2 slices whole wheat bread
2 oz of sliced turkey (low sodium or home roasted turkey)
1/8 cup Cabot® Reduced Fat Sharp Cheddar Cheese, shredded
1/8 medium avocado, thinly sliced
1/2 cup spring mix salad
1/4 medium tomato, sliced
1 tbsp light olive oil mayonnaise
1 tsp mustard
jalapeño pepper slices or pickle slices optional

Toast the bread. Spread light olive oil mayonnaise and mustard on both slices of bread. Layer bottom half of bread with spring mix, tomatoes, avocado, and peppers or pickles (optional.) Layer top half with shredded cheese and slice turkey (cold or slightly heated in skillet sprayed with cooking spray). Press two sides together lightly and serve.

Nutritional Facts: Nutritional information based on one (1) serving or 1 sandwich.
Calories: 259 | **Fat:** 10g | **Fiber:** 7g | **Carbs:** 28g | **Protein:** 24g | **Sugar:** 4g

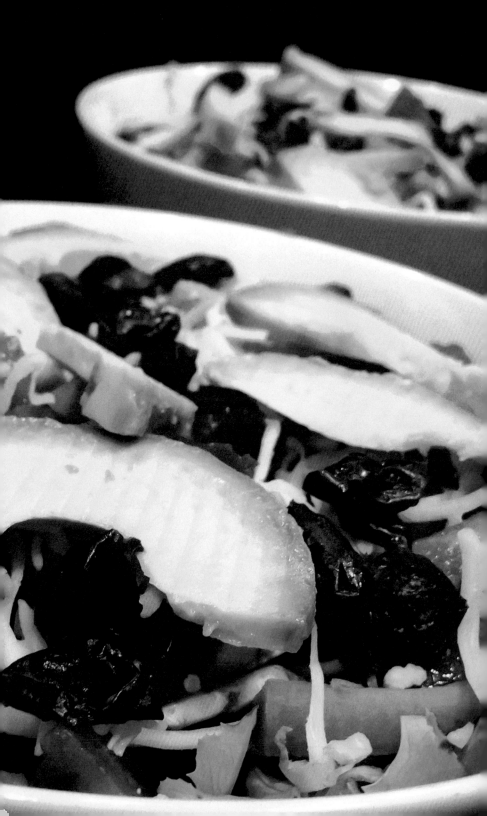

cranberry avocado salad

Servings: 2

3 cups baby spinach, arugula, field greens
2/3 ripe avocado, peeled, seeded, and sliced
1/8 cup dried cranberries
1/2 cup tomato, chopped
1/2 cup mushrooms, sliced
1/4 cup low fat cheddar/colby cheese
1/2 cup carrots, shredded
Balasamic Vinaigrette Dressing

Place greens in a large bowl. Add tomatoes, carrots, mushrooms, & cheese. Toss salad gently, combining ingredients. Top with avocado slices. Sprinkle lightly with salt and freshly ground black pepper.

Top with Balasamic Vinaigrette Dressing or dressing of choice. Enjoy!

Nutritional Facts: Nutritional information based on one (1) serving.
Calories: 196 | **Fat:** 10g | **Fiber:** 8g | **Carbs:** 19g | **Protein:** 9g | **Sugar:** 8g

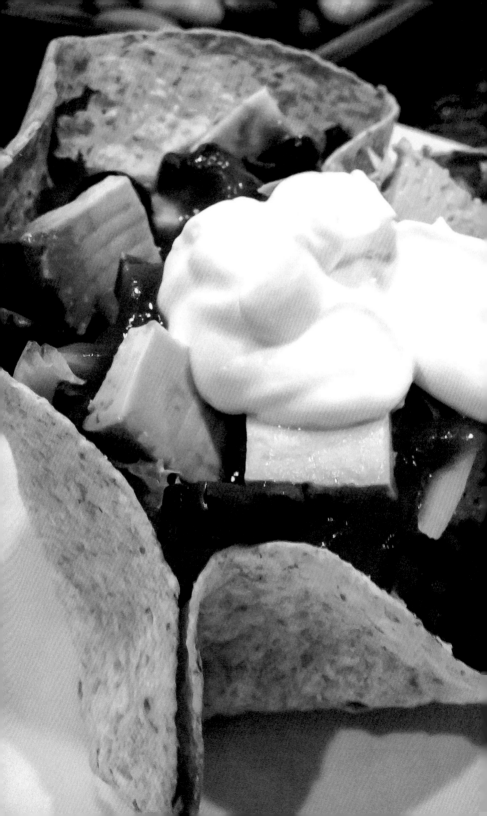

fish taco salad

Servings: 4

4 whole wheat tortillas (8 inch)
4 tilapia filets, sauteed & chopped
1 tbsp extra virgin olive oil
1 tbsp smart balance® light with flaxseed oil
1 1/2 cup arugula, chopped
1 large tomato, chopped or fresh salsa *(recipe on pg. 151)*
1/2 cup black olives, sliced
1/2 avocado, cubed
1/2 cup low fat cheddar cheese
4 tbsp light sour cream or greek yogurt

Taco Bowls: Heat oven to 425°F. Crumble 4 sheets of foil to make 4 (3-inch) balls; place on baking sheet. Top each with 1 tortilla; spray with cooking spray. Bake 6 to 8 min. or until tortillas are golden brown. (Tortillas will drape over balls as they bake to form shells.) Set aside.

Season tilapia filets with salt & pepper (or seasonings of choice). In large skillet, coat with 1 tbsp olive oil and 1 tbsp Smart Balance® Light. Heat skillet on medium heat. Place tilapia filets in skillet & sauté on both sides until done. Remove from skillet, crumble or rough chop. Set aside.

Fill tortilla shells with crumbled tilapia filets, arugula, diced tomatoes/ fresh salsa, black olives, avocados, cheese. Top with light sour cream. Try drizzling with your favorite taco sauce or balsamic vinegar. Enjoy!

Nutritional Facts: Nutritional information based on one (1) serving or 1 taco salad.
Calories: 347 | **Fat:** 16g | **Fiber:** 6g | **Carbs:** 30g | **Protein:** 23g | **Sugar:** 6g

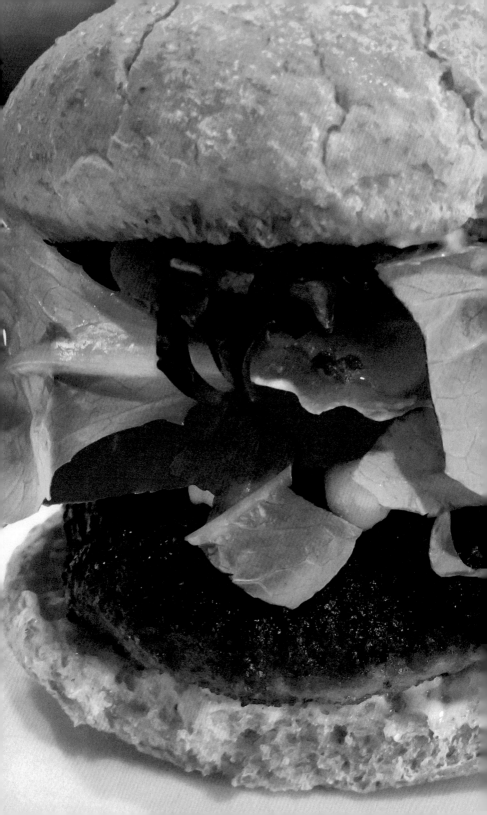

turkey burger

Servings: 8

2 lbs lean ground turkey
1 onion, chopped fine
1 tsp garlic powder
2 tbsp extra virgin olive oil
2 tbsp Worcestershire sauce
1/2 cup panko crumbs
1 tbsp parsley
1 tsp Goya® adobo
1 tsp cayenne pepper
1 tsp black pepper

8 whole wheat buns
1/4 cup Cabot® Reduced
Fat Sharp Cheddar Cheese,
shredded
1/4 medium avocado, thinly
sliced
1 cup spring mix salad, chopped
1/4 medium tomato, sliced
1 tbsp light olive oil mayonnaise
1 tsp mustard
pickle slices (optional)

In large bowl, mix ground turkey, chopped onion, panko crumbs, Worcestershire sauce, parsley, pepper, adobo, cayenne pepper, and garlic powder. Form into 8 (4oz) patties.

In skillet over medium heat, add olive oil and cook patties, turning once. Cook burgers to an internal temperature of 180°F. Remove and set aside.

To Assemble Burgers:
Dress whole wheat buns with mayonnaise, mustard, cheese, spring mix, tomato, avocado, and pickles. Serve with roasted sweet potato fries, kale chips, 1 serving of your favorite chips, or steamed vegetable.

Nutritional Facts: Nutritional information based on one (1) serving or 1 dressed burger.
Calories: 436 | **Fat:** 20g | **Fiber:** 5g | **Carbs:** 36g | **Protein:** 31g | **Sugar:** 4g

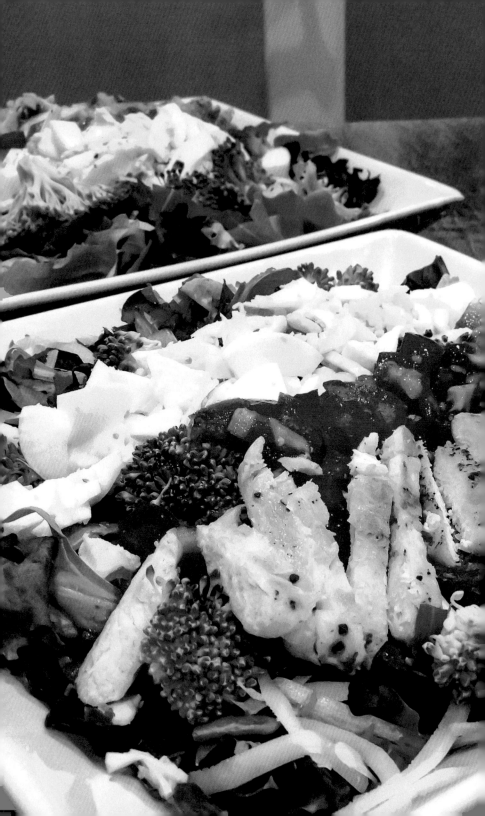

chicken broccoli salad

Servings: 2

3 cups baby spinach, arugula, field greens
4 oz boneless skinless chicken breast, pan seared & sliced.
2 hard boiled eggs, chopped
1 cup tomato, chopped
1 cup broccoli florets
1/4 cup low fat cheddar/colby cheese
Balasamic Vinaigrette Dressing

Season both sides of chicken breast with sea salt and black pepper. Place seasoned chicken breasts inside ziploc bag. Use meat tenderizer and pound chicken breasts until thin. In large skillet, over medium-high heat, add olive oil and cook chicken breasts for about 8 minutes on each side or until juices run clear. Set aside. Cut into slices.

Place greens in a large bowl. Add broccoli florets, eggs, tomatoes, cheese, & chicken slices.

Top with Balasamic Vinaigrette Dressing or dressing of choice. Enjoy!

Nutritional Facts: Nutritional information based on one (1) serving.
Calories: 288 | **Fat:** 15g | **Fiber:** 4g | **Carbs:** 10g | **Protein:** 28g | **Sugar:** 3g

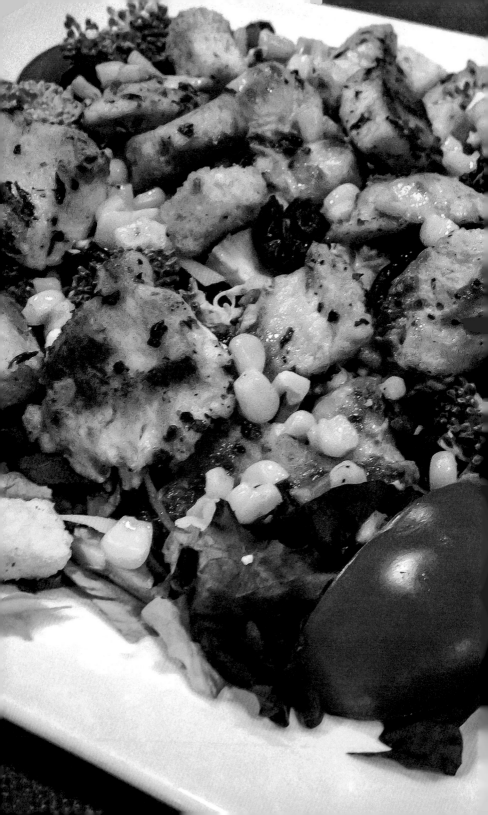

southwest chicken salad

Servings: 2

3 cups baby spinach, arugula, field greens
4 oz boneless skinless chicken breast, pan seared & cubed.
1 tbsp extra virgin olive oil (pan searing)
1/2 cup yellow corn, steamed or steam fresh packaged corn
2 tomatoes, quartered
1 cup broccoli florets
1 tbsp dried cranberries or craisins
1/2 medium avocado, cut in bite size pieces
1/4 cup low fat cheddar/colby cheese
seasoned croutons optional (1 serving according to product label)
Balasamic Vinaigrette Dressing

Season both sides of chicken breast with 1 tsp chili powder, paprika, garlic powder, parsley, sea salt and black pepper. Place seasoned chicken breasts inside ziploc bag. Use meat tenderizer and pound chicken breasts until thin. In large skillet, over medium-high heat, add olive oil and cook chicken breasts for about 8 minutes on each side or until juices run clear. Set aside. Cut chicken into cubes.

Place greens in a large bowl. Add broccoli florets, corn, cranberries/craisins, avocado, tomatoes, cheese, & chicken.

Top with Garlic Vinaigrette Dressing or dressing of choice. Enjoy!

Nutritional Facts: Nutritional information based on one (1) serving.
Calories: 326 | **Fat:** 17g | **Fiber:** 7g | **Carbs:** 27g | **Protein:** 21g | **Sugar:** 7g

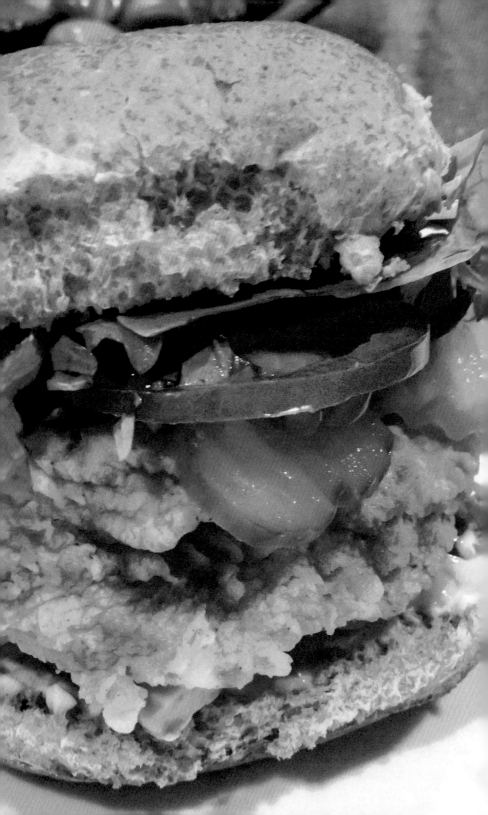

crispy chicken sandwich

Servings: 4

2 - 4oz boneless/skinless
chicken breasts
1 tsp Tony Chachere's® Creole
Seasoning
1-2 cups panko crumbs, crushed
1 tbsp extra virgin olive oil

4 whole wheat buns
1/4 cup Cabot® Reduced
Fat Sharp Cheddar Cheese,
shredded
1 cup spring mix salad, chopped
1/4 medium tomato, sliced
1 tbsp light olive oil mayonnaise
1 tsp mustard
pickle slices optional

Preheat oven to 400°F. Line cookie sheet with foil. Spray with non-stick cooking spray. Place panko crumbs in shallow dish. Set aside.

Coat chicken breast with olive oil. Season both sides of chicken breast with Tony Chachere's® creole seasoning. Place seasoned chicken breasts inside ziploc bag. Use meat tenderizer and pound chicken breasts until thin. Cut each breast in half. Lightly coat each side in crushed panko crumbs. Place on cookie sheet. Bake for 15-18 minutes, turning once, until juice of chicken is clear and coating is golden brown.

To Assemble Chicken Sandwiches:
Dress whole wheat buns with mayonnaise, mustard, cheese, spring mix, tomato, avocado, and pickles. Serve with roasted sweet potato fries, kale chips, 1 serving of your favorite chips, or steamed vegetable.

Enjoy!

Nutritional Facts: Nutritional information based on one (1) serving or 1 chicken sandwich.
Calories: 338 | **Fat:** 12g | **Fiber:** 5g | **Carbs:** 40g | **Protein:** 21g | **Sugar:** 4g

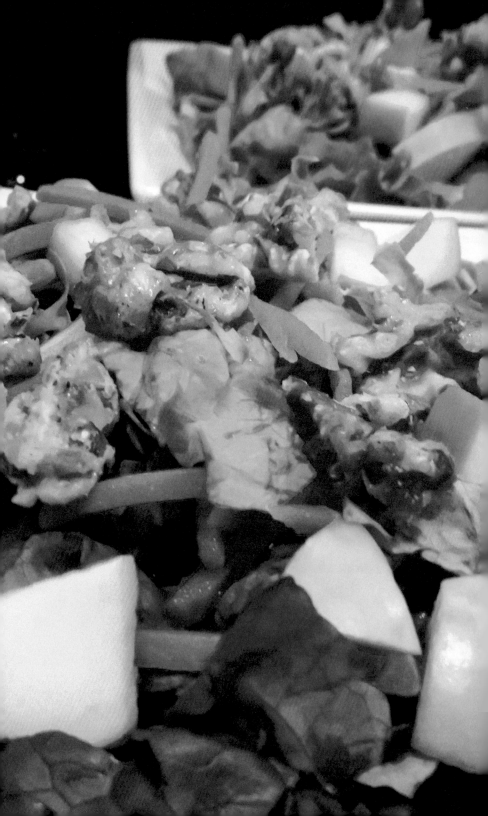

apple walnut salad

Servings: 2

3 cups baby spinach, arugula, field greens
1 small green apple, chopped
1/2 cup shredded carrots
1/4 cup walnuts, lightly toasted
Balasamic Vinaigrette Dressing

Preheat oven to 350°F. Place walnuts in single layer on cooking sheet. Bake for 8-10 minutes, until lightly toasted

Place greens in a large bowl. Add carrots and apples. Sprinkle with walnuts. Top with Balasamic Vinaigrette Dressing or dressing of choice.

Enjoy!

Nutritional Facts: Nutritional information based on one (1) serving.
Calories: 160 | **Fat:** 10g | **Fiber:** 5g | **Carbs:** 15g | **Protein:** 5g | **Sugar:** 7g

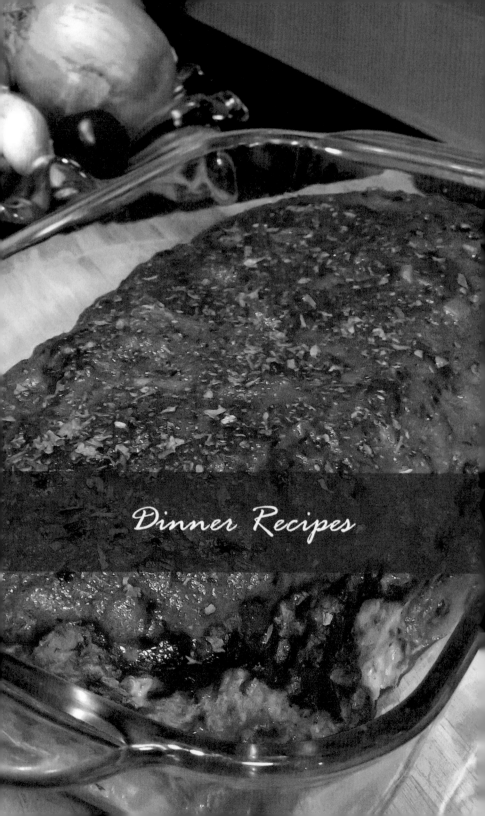

Dinner Recipes

dinner tip

Dinner is beyond just having a healthier, end-of-the-day meal. Dinner is about gathering with your family after a long day to reconnect, communicate, and share the secret ingredient you should be putting in all of your foods...LOVE.

Always include lean proteins, vegetables, and whole grains. Most importantly, enjoy dinner with your family.

DO NOT SKIP DINNER!

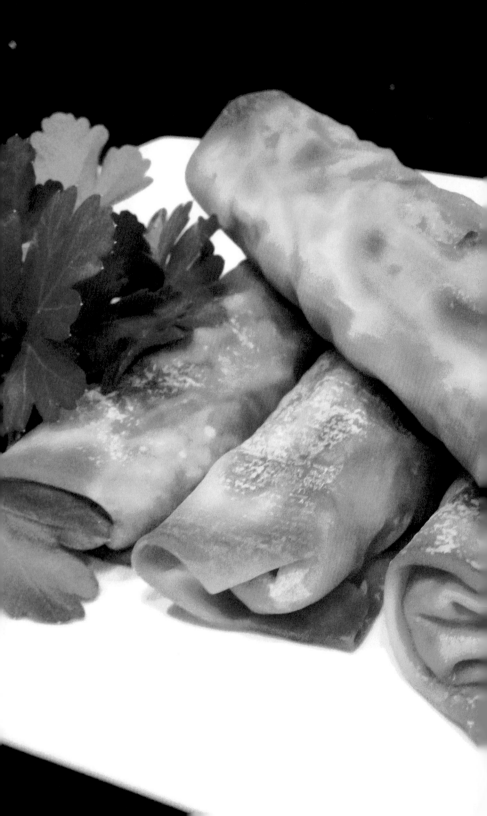

baked egg rolls

Servings: 16-20

2 cups cabbage, shredded
1 cup carrots, shredded
1 cup bean sprouts
1/4 cup bell pepper, chopped
2 cloves minced garlic
2 cups cooked chicken breast, chopped
16 egg roll wrappers
nonstick cooking spray

Egg Roll Sauce:
4 tsp cornstarch
1 tbsp water
1 tbsp light soy sauce
1 tsp extra virgin olive oil
1 tsp Splenda® Brown Sugar
pinch cayenne pepper

Preheat oven to 425°F. Lightly grease a baking sheet. Coat chicken breast with olive oil. Sprinkle sea salt & pepper on both sides of chicken breast. Place chicken breasts inside ziploc bag. Use meat tenderizer and pound chicken until thin. Cook in skillet and set aside. In same skillet, cook and stir cabbage, carrots, bean sprouts, green pepper, and garlic until vegetables are crisp. Cut up chicken & add to cabbage mixture. Mix in sauce. Cook until heated through.

Sauce: Combine cornstarch, water, soy sauce, 1 teaspoon oil, brown sugar, and cayenne in a small bowl; stir into chicken mixture. Bring to a boil over high heat and stir, cooking until sauce is thickened, about 2 minutes; remove from heat.

To make each egg roll: Spoon 1/4 cup chicken mixture on the bottom third of one egg roll wrapper. Fold sides toward center and roll tightly; place seam side down on baking sheet. Repeat with remaining filling and wrappers. Spray top of egg rolls with nonstick cooking spray. Bake in preheated oven until lightly browned, 10-15 minutes. Enjoy!

Nutritional Facts: Nutritional information based on one (1) serving or 1 egg roll.
Calories: 108 | **Fat:** 2g | **Fiber:** 1g | **Carbs:** 16g | **Protein:** 6g | **Sugar:** 2g

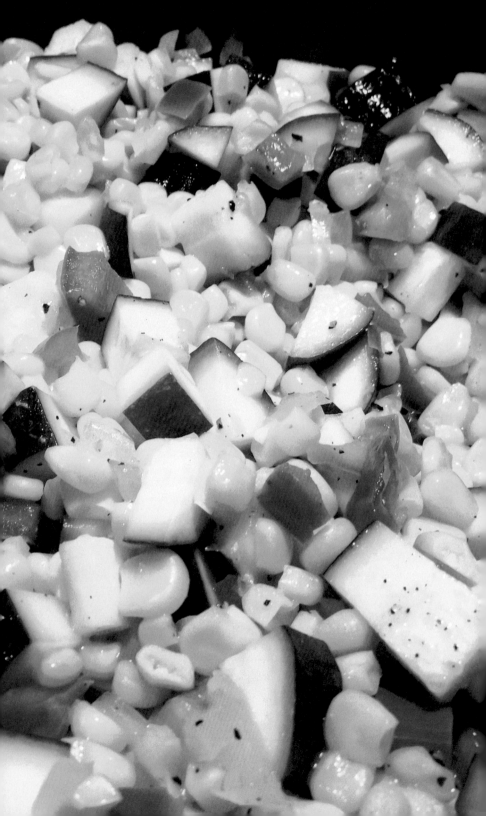

sweet corn succotash

Servings: 8

4 cups sweet corn
2 cups green zucchini, chopped
1 medium bell pepper, chopped
1 medium sweet onion, chopped
3 garlic cloves, peeled and chopped
2 tbsp extra virgin olive oil
sea salt and pepper

Heat the olive oil in a saute pan over medium heat. Add the onion, and garlic. Saute until onions become slightly translucent. Add the bellpepper and saute for two more minutes. Add the zucchini and corn, cooking until veggies soften. Fold in the cilantro or fresh parsley. Season to taste with sea salt and pepper. Enjoy!

Nutritional Facts: Nutritional information based on one (1) serving or 1/2 cup.
Calories: 115 | **Fat:** 5g | **Fiber:** 4g | **Carbs:** 16g | **Protein:** 3g | **Sugar:** 7g

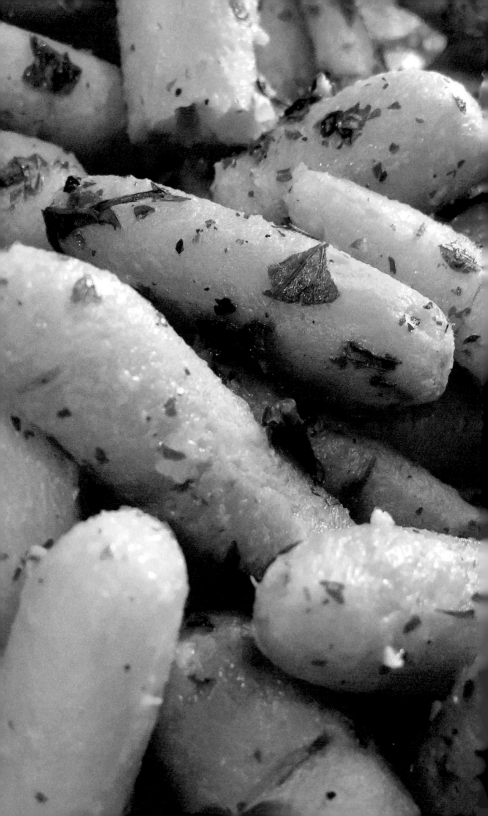

glazed carrots

Servings: 8

2 - 16 oz packaged of baby carrots
2 tbsp butter, unsalted
2 tbsp parsley
1/4 tsp Splenda® or sweetener of choice
sea salt and black pepper

Add carrots to 3-quart saucepan and cover with water. Add salt and pepper. Bring to boil; reduce heat. Slightly cover (allow steam to escape) and cook for about 10 minutes or until tender preference. Drain and return to saucepan. Add butter, sweetener, and parsley. Simmer over low heat for about 5 minutes, stirring constantly until well blended.

Enjoy!

Nutritional Facts: Nutritional information based on one (1) serving or 1/2 cup.
Calories: 73 | **Fat:** 3g | **Fiber:** 3g | **Carbs:** 8g | **Protein:** 1g | **Sugar:** 7g

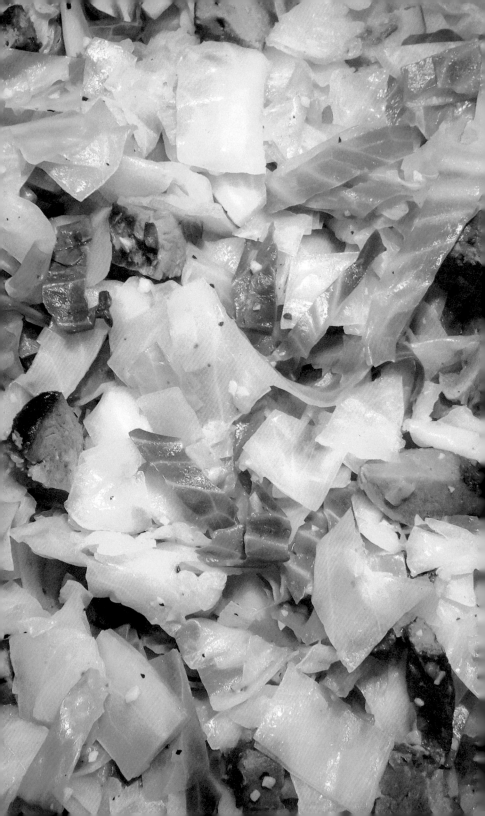

sautéed cabbage

Servings: 8

1 large head of cabbage, sliced or chopped
1 8oz pkg Turkey Tasso*, cubed
1 medium onion, chopped
3 cloves garlic, minced
1 tbsp extra virgin olive oil
1/4 cup low sodium chicken stock or water
sea salt and black pepper
cayenne pepper

Cut the cabbage in half and, with the cut-side down, slice it as thinly as possible around the core.

Heat olive oil in skillet. Add onions and garlic and sauté lightly. Add cabbage in batches until all cabbage has been cooked down in skillet. Add 1/4 cup of chicken stock or water. Stir. Add turkey tasso, cayenne pepper, salt and black pepper. Be sure to taste cabbage before adding salt when using stock. *(Stock tends to have enough sodium for your foods).* Saute for 15 to 20 minutes, stirring occasionally, until the cabbage is tender.

Enjoy as side dish or with Brown/Jasmine Rice.

Substitute Turkey Tasso with turkey ham or turkey sausage.

Nutritional Facts: Nutritional information based on one (1) serving or 1/2 cup.
Calories: 95 | **Fat:** 3g | **Fiber:** 5g | **Carbs:** 10g | **Protein:** 9g | **Sugar:** 5g

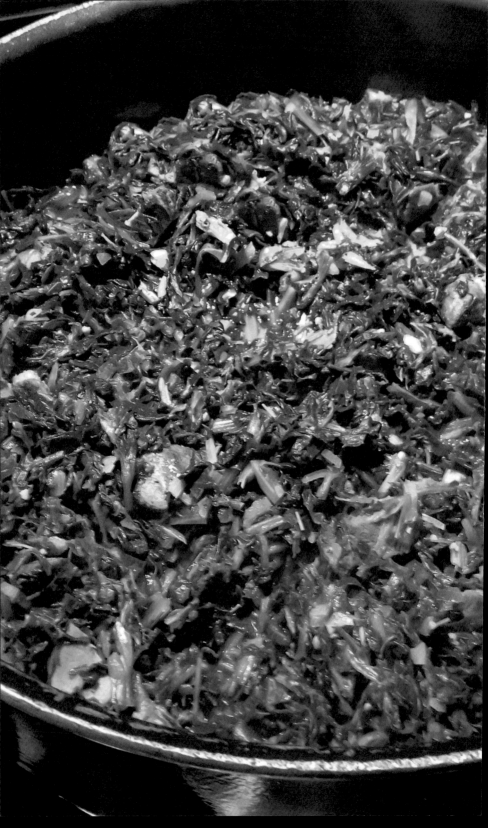

mixed greens

Servings: 10-12

1 16oz pkg Collard Greens, frozen
1 16oz pkg Mustard Greens, frozen
1 16oz pkg Turnip Greens, frozen
1 16oz pkg Spinach, frozen
1lb Turkey Tasso, cubed*
1 medium onion, chopped

2 cloves garlic, minced
2 tbsp extra virgin olive oil
2-4 cups low sodium chicken stock or water
salt and black pepper
cayenne pepper
2 tbsp white vinegar

Heat olive oil in large skillet. Add onions and garlic and sauté lightly. Add turkey tasso and continue sautéing for 5 minutes. Add frozen greens and 1-2 cups of chicken stock. Season with black pepper & cayenne pepper. Taste before adding salt. *(Stock tends to salt your dishes without needing to add additional salt. Add additional stock based on tenderness and preferred liquid consistency in greens.)*

Bring to a boil, reduce heat to a simmer, and cook until the greens are tender, stirring occasionally, 30-45 minutes. Enjoy!

Substitute Turkey Tasso with turkey ham, turkey sausage, or omit meat.

Nutritional Facts: Nutritional information based on one (1) serving or 1 cup.
Calories: 103 | **Fat:** 3g | **Fiber:** 3g | **Carbs:** 7g | **Protein:** 8g | **Sugar:** 0g

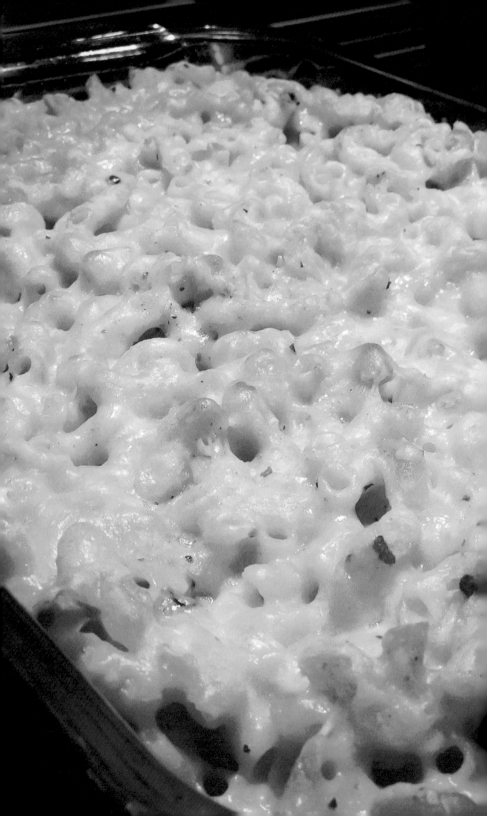

baked macaroni

Servings: 12-14

1lb (16oz package) whole wheat elbow pasta, cooked
2-2 1/2 cups Cabot® Reduced Fat Sharp Cheddar Cheese
2-2 1/2 cups Unsweetened Almond Milk
2 tbsp unsalted butter or coconut oil
1 egg
1/4 cup bread crumbs (optional topping)
sea salt and black pepper

Preheat oven to 350°F. Spray baking or casserole dish with non-stick cooking spray. Set aside. In a bowl, mix together the egg, 1 1/2cups almond milk, salt and pepper. Add butter to large pot and add cooked macaroni. Mix well to coat macaroni with butter. Add milk mixture to macaroni and sprinkle about 1/2 cup of cheese. Mix well.

Pour half of the macaroni into baking dish. Sprinkle with 1/2 cup of cheese. Pour remaining macaroni into baking dish. Top with remaining cheese and 1/2 cup of almond milk. Sprinkle top with bread crumbs. Bake, uncovered, until the top is golden and cheese is melted. Enjoy!

Nutritional Facts: Nutritional information based on one (1) serving or 1/3-1/2 cup.
Calories: 202 | **Fat:** 7g | **Fiber:** 2g | **Carbs:** 20g | **Protein:** 15g | **Sugar:** 1g

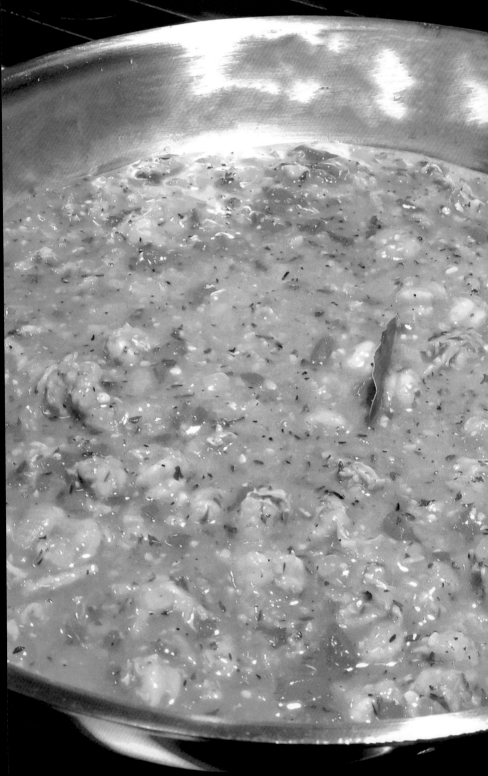

crawfish etouffee

Servings: 6

1lb peeled crawfish tails
1 medium onion, chopped
1 medium bell pepper, chopped
4 garlic cloves, minced
2 bay leaves
2 tbsp butter
2 tbsp extra virgin olive oil
1 tbsp flour
1 cup seafood stock
pinch cayenne pepper
sea salt and black pepper
2 tbsp chopped parsley

In large saute pan, melt butter and olive oil over medium heat. Add onions, garlic, and bell pepper. Saute until vegetables are soft. Add the flour and brown with seasonings to create a simple roux. Add seafood stock gradually until etouffee thins slightly. Add crawfish tails, cayenne pepper and bay leaves. Add salt and pepper. Cook for 15 minutes, stirring occasionally. Sauce will thicken. You can add additional stock based on your preference.

Stir in parsley and continue cooking for 5 minutes. Serve over jasmine rice or brown rice.

Nutritional Facts: Nutritional information based on one (1) serving or 1/3-1/2 cup.
Calories: 145 | **Fat:** 9g | **Fiber:** 1g | **Carbs:** 5g | **Protein:** 11g | **Sugar:** 2g

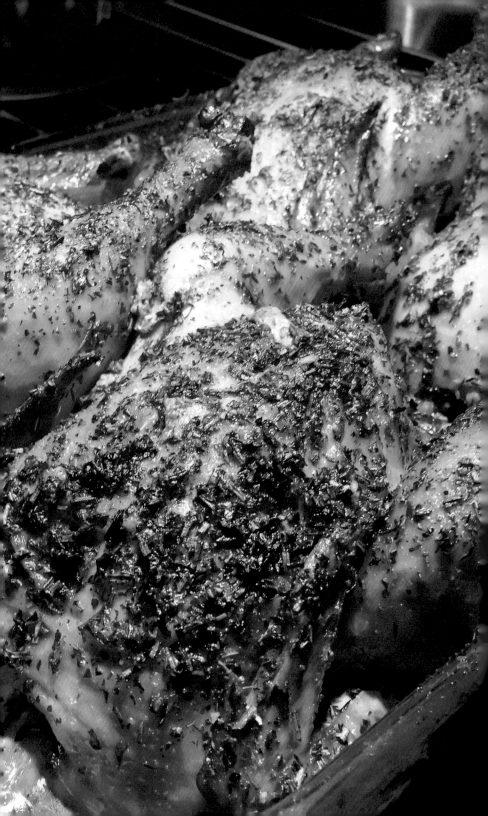

apple thyme roasted chicken

Servings: 8-10

3-5 lb whole chicken
3 tbsp extra virgin olive oil
1 medium sweet onion, cubed
1 medium red or green apple, cubed
2 tbsp thyme
2 tbsp rosemary
2 tbsp sage
sea salt and pepper

Preheat oven to 425°F. Chop up your herbs and set aside. Mix salt and pepper in small dish, set aside. Make sure the outside of the chicken is patted dry with a paper towel. Before we coat the outside of the chicken, we need to fill the cavity. Drizzle a little olive oil inside the cavity. Sprinkle cavity with a few pinches of your salt/pepper mixture and herbs. Stuff the chicken with your cubed onion and apples.

Drizzle the olive oil on the whole chicken and underneath skin. Sprinkle herb mixture, salt/pepper and rub, rub, rub until it is well coated. Place chicken on roasting pan or 13×9-inch baking dish. Bake for 1 hour until golden brown. *Tip: Baste your chicken with chicken drippings in bottom of baking pan every 15 minutes.* (meat thermometer should read 185°F in the thigh meat)

Once the chicken has roasted, let it rest for 10-15 minutes. This will allow the juices of the chicken redistribute & ensure your chicken is moist & delicious.

We always slice the chicken breast so we can measure smaller portions and add to our salads during the week. Enjoy!

Nutritional Facts: Nutritional information based on one (1) serving or 2-4 oz.
Calories: 140 | **Fat:** 10g | **Fiber:** 1g | **Carbs:** 4g | **Protein:** 8g | **Sugar:** 2g

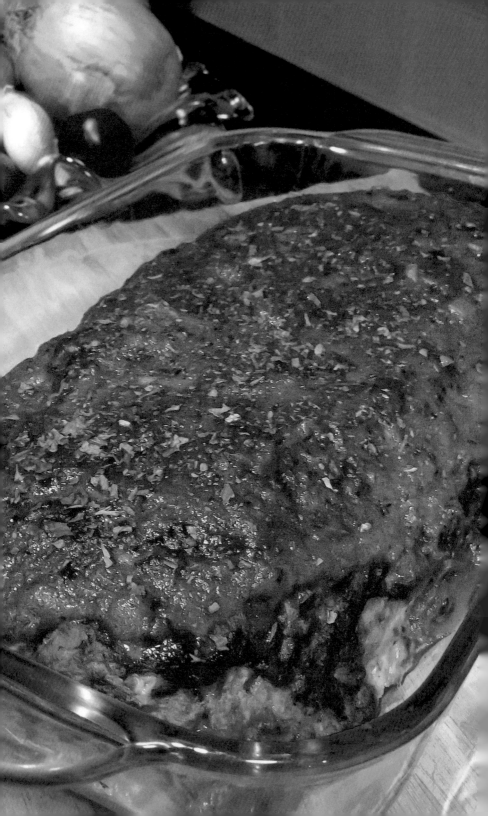

turkey meatloaf

Servings: 10-12

2 ¹⁄² lbs lean ground turkey
1 onion, chopped fine
3 cloves garlic, minced
2 tbsp extra virgin olive oil
1/2 cup Egg Beaters®
2 tbsp Worcestershire sauce
1/2-3/4 cup panko bread crumbs
3/4 cup tomato sauce
1/2 tsp basil
1/2 tsp parsley
sea salt and pepper

Heat oven to 350°F. Heat extra virgin olive oil in a small skillet over medium-high heat. Add onion and garlic; cook 5 minutes, stirring occasionally. Transfer mixture to a large bowl; cool 5 minutes.

Add ground turkey, panko bread crumbs, egg, ¼ cup tomato sauce, Worcestershire sauce, parsley, basil, salt and pepper, if desired to turkey mixture; mix well. Press & mold into 13 x 9-inch baking pan. Spread remaining tomato sauce over top.

Bake 1 hour or until the internal temperature of meatloaf is well-done, 185°F. as measured by a meat thermometer. Let meatloaf rest a few minutes before slicing. Enjoy!

Nutritional Facts: Nutritional information based on one (1) serving or 2-4 oz..
Calories: 233 | **Fat:** 11g | **Fiber:** 1g | **Carbs:** 7g | **Protein:** 23g | **Sugar:** 2g

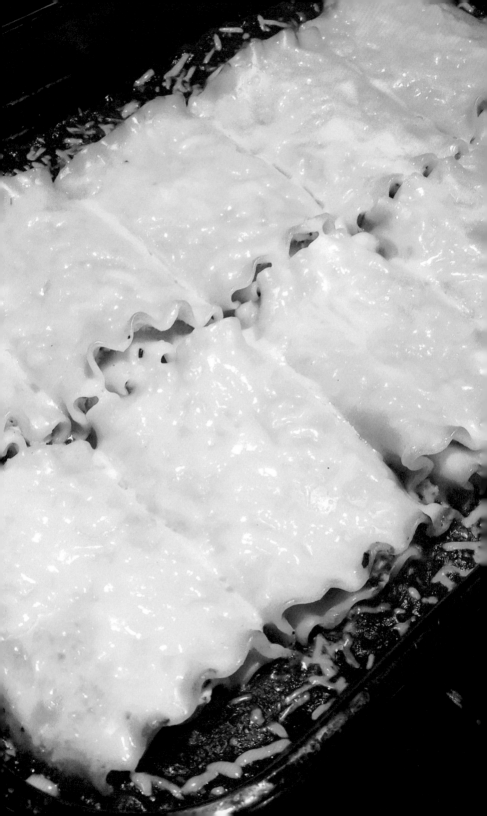

zucchini lasagne rolls

Servings: 10

1/2 lb (10 strips) whole wheat lasagne noodles, cooked
3 cups tomato sauce
3 cups zucchini, peeled & grated
2 tbsp extra virgin olive oil
$1^{1/2}$ cups sweet onion, chopped
2 cloves garlic, minced
1 tsp dried basil
1 tsp dried oregano
1/2 cup low fat cheddar cheese
2 cups light ricotta cheese
sea salt and pepper

Preheat oven to 375°F. Heat olive oil in a skillet. Add onions and garlic, and cook until soft and translucent. Be sure to stir regularly so you don't burn your garlic. Set aside and cool. In large bowl, add ricotta cheese, basil, oregano, zucchini, and cooled onion mixture. Add salt and pepper. Mix well.

Assemble Lasagne Rolls:
Lay one lasagne noodle strip flat on working surface. Spread 1/4 cup of cheese mixture evenly along the strip from end to end. Roll up the strip and place it in 13 x 9 baking dish. (Be sure to spray dish). Continue until all noodles are rolled and placed in dish. Pour tomato sauce around the sides of each lasagne rolls. Do not put any sauce on the top of the rolls. Sprinkle cheese on top. Cover dish with foil and bake for about 20-25 minutes or until hot & bubbly. If using Parmesan cheese, add cheese after rolls have baked; right before serving. Enjoy!

Nutritional Facts: Nutritional information based on one (1) serving or 1 roll.
Calories: 261 | **Fat:** 10g | **Fiber:** 3g | **Carbs:** 32g | **Protein:** 13g | **Sugar:** 9g

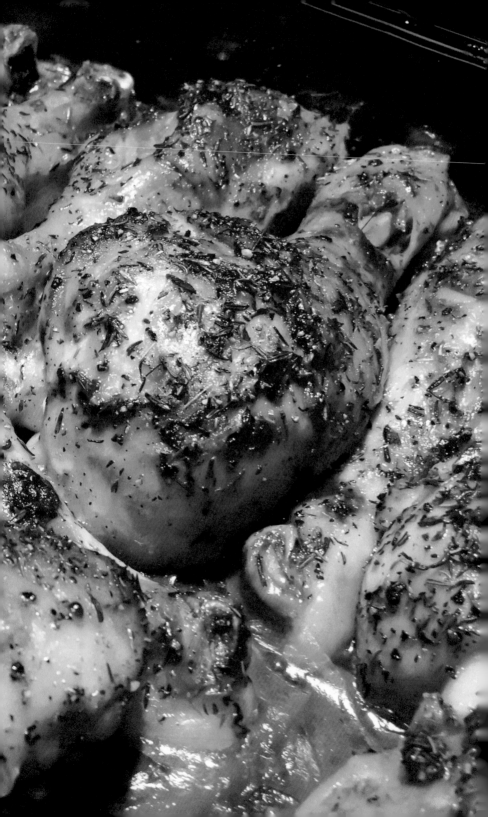

herb roasted chicken

Servings: 16

16 chicken drumsticks
2 tbsp extra virgin olive oil
2 tbsp thyme
2 tbsp rosemary
2 tbsp parsley
1/4 cup water or low sodium chicken stock *(enough to cover the bottom)*
sea salt and pepper

Preheat oven to 425°F. Coat the chicken with olive oil and season with thyme, rosemary, salt and pepper. Place chicken drumsticks in 13x9 baking dish. Add water.

Bake for 30-45 minutes, or until a meat thermometer reads 185°F.

Enjoy!

Nutritional Facts: Nutritional information based on one (1) serving or 1 drumstick.
Calories: 91 | **Fat:** 6g | **Fiber:** 0g | **Carbs:** 0g | **Protein:** 9g | **Sugar:** 0g

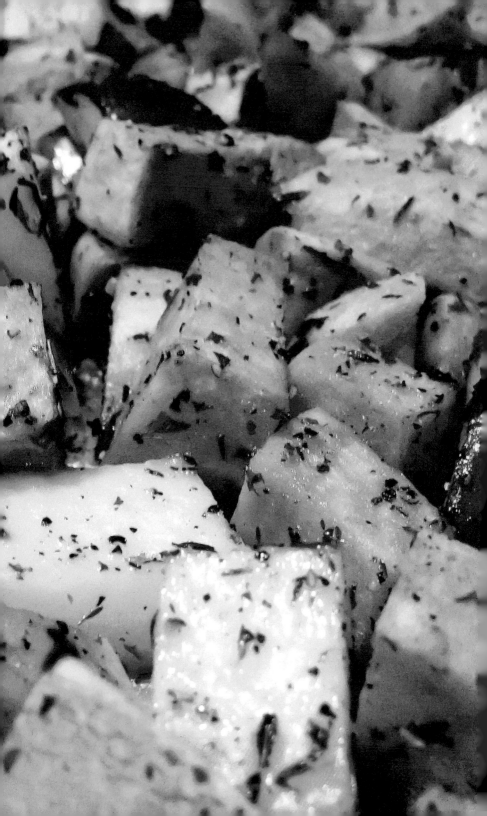

herb roasted sweet & red potatoes

Servings: 6-8

4 medium sweet potatoes, peeled, cut into 1 1/2-inch thick cubes
3 small red potatoes, cut into 1 1/2-inch thick cubes
2 tablespoon extra virgin olive oil
1 tablespoon thyme
1 tablespoon parsley
sea salt & black pepper

Preheat oven to 425°F. In large mixing bowl, combine all ingredients and toss. Arrange potato pieces in a single layer on heavyweight rimmed baking sheet or in 13×9-inch baking dish. Place on middle rack of oven and roast until tender and slightly browned, about 40 minutes.

Enjoy!

Nutritional Facts: Nutritional information based on one (1) serving or 1/2 cup.
Calories: 125 | **Fat:** 4g | **Fiber:** 3g | **Carbs:** 25g | **Protein:** 2g | **Sugar:** 4g

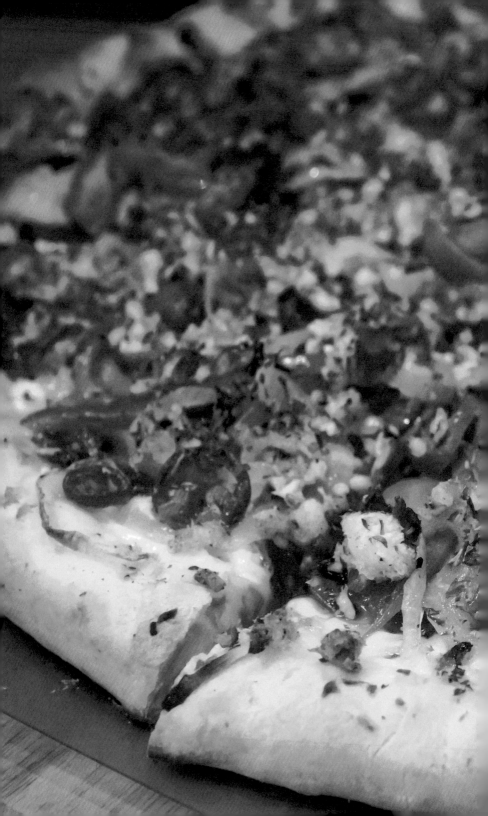

sautéed tilapia & vegetable pizza

Servings: 6-8

12" Whole Wheat Thin Pizza Crust
3/4 cup tomato sauce
2 - 4oz tilapia filets, sautéed
1/2 cup sliced jalapeno peppers
1/4-1/2 cup sliced black olives
1 cup sliced mushrooms
1/2 onion, sliced thin

1/2 green bell pepper, sliced thin
1 tbsp parsley
2 cloves fresh garlic, chopped
2 cups low fat mozzarella cheese
2 tbsp extra virgin olive oil
1 tbsp Smart Balance® light
sea salt & pepper to taste

Preheat oven to 425°F. Season tilapia filets with salt & pepper. In large skillet, coat with 1 tbsp olive oil and 1 tbsp Smart Balance® Light. Heat skillet on medium heat. Place tilapia filets in skillet & sauté on both sides until done. Remove from skillet and set aside. In same skillet, combine all veggies except jalapeno peppers and black olives, season with salt and pepper, sauté for 5min. Remove from skillet and set aside to cool. Remember, the veggies will cook in the oven.

Brush the crust with olive oil and spread the tomato sauce over pizza crust leaving a 1" border. Sprinkle half the cheese around crust. Arrange sautéed vegetables in a single layer. Add jalapeno peppers and black olives. Add crumbled tilapia. Add remaining cheese to top of pizza. Sprinkle entire pizza with remaining olive oil. Place in oven and bake for about 8 – 10 minutes or until cheese is melted. Remove from oven and let set for 5 minutes. Sprinkle parsley over the top. Enjoy!

Nutritional Facts: Nutritional information based on one (1) serving or 1 slice.
Calories: 200 | **Fat:** 11g | **Fiber:** 2g | **Carbs:** 10g | **Protein:** 15g | **Sugar:** 3g

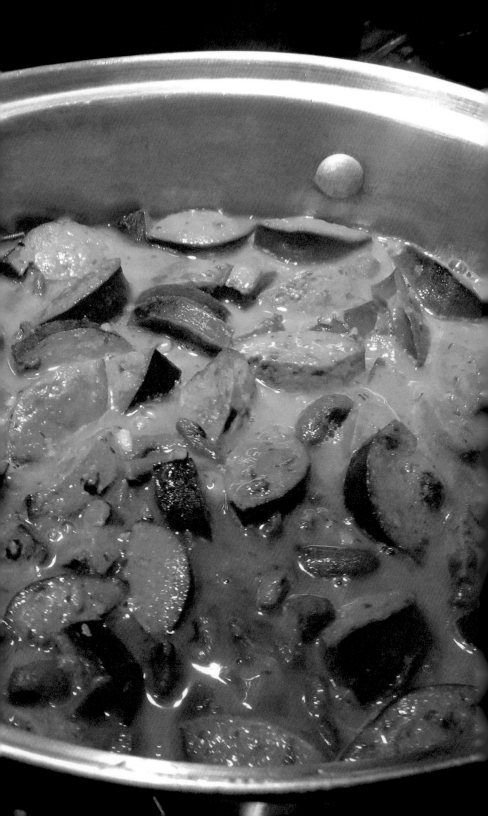

red beans and jasmine rice

Servings: 6-8

1lb red kidney beans (any beans)
1 8oz pkg turkey tasso*
2 tbsp extra virgin olive oil
1 large onion, chopped
1 green bell pepper, chopped
4 garlic cloves, chopped
10 cups of water or low sodium

chicken stock
4 bay leaves
1 tsp cayenne pepper
2 tbsp parsley
sea salt and black pepper
2 cups Jasmine rice

Rinse beans and pick out all the bad beans. Put beans in large pot. Add 10 cups of water or stock, bay leaves, and cook on low heat. In a skillet, heat olive oil over medium heat. Cook tasso or turkey smoke sausage for 5 minutes. Remove from skillet and set aside. Add onions, garlic, and bell pepper to same skillet and saute seasonings for 5 minutes or until slightly translucent. Add cooked seasoning, cayenne pepper, black pepper, salt (to taste) to beans. Stir and cover.

Bring to a boil and then reduce heat to medium-low. Simmer for 2-2 1/2 hours. Add parsley, smoke sausage or turkey tasso and continue to simmer for approximately 30 minutes.

Prepare Jasmine rice according to directions. Serve beans over jasmine rice. You can substitute with brown rice or enjoy with no rice at all.

Substitute Turkey Tasso with turkey ham, turkey sausage, sauteed chicken breasts, cubed, or omit meat.

Nutritional Facts: Nutritional information based on one (1) serving or 1 cup of beans.
Calories: 347 | **Fat:** 7g | **Fiber:** 16g | **Carbs:** 46g | **Protein:** 24g | **Sugar:** 5g

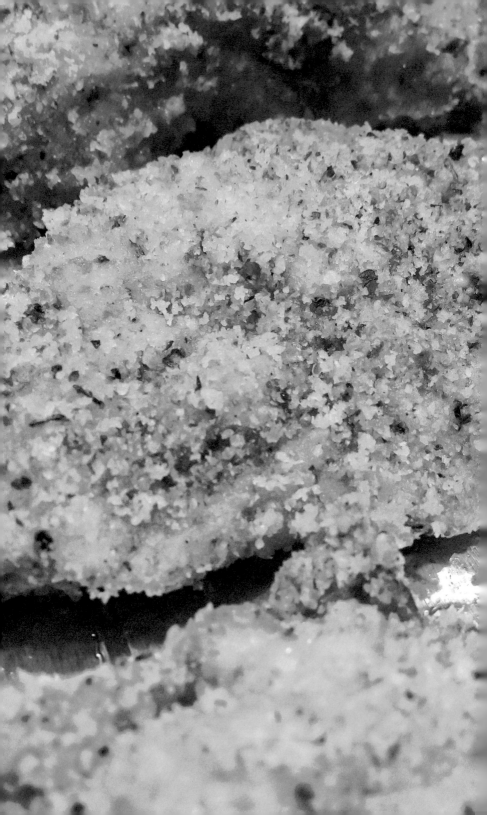

baked parmesan chicken

Servings: 12

6 skinless, boneless chicken breasts, split in half (12 breast)
2 tbsp extra virgin olive oil
3 clove garlic, minced
2 cups panko italian bread crumbs, crushed
2 tbsp sweet basil
sea salt and black pepper

Preheat oven to 350°F. Lightly grease a 9x13 inch baking dish. In a bowl, blend the olive oil and garlic. In a separate bowl, mix the bread crumbs, basil, and pepper. Dip each chicken breast in the oil mixture, then in the bread crumb mixture. Arrange the coated chicken breasts in the prepared baking dish, and top with any remaining bread crumb mixture.

Bake 30 minutes in the preheated oven, or until chicken is no longer pink and juices run clear. Enjoy!

Nutritional Facts: Nutritional information based on one (1) serving or 1 breast.
Calories: 146 | **Fat:** 5g | **Fiber:** 1g | **Carbs:** 4g | **Protein:** 22g | **Sugar:** 0g

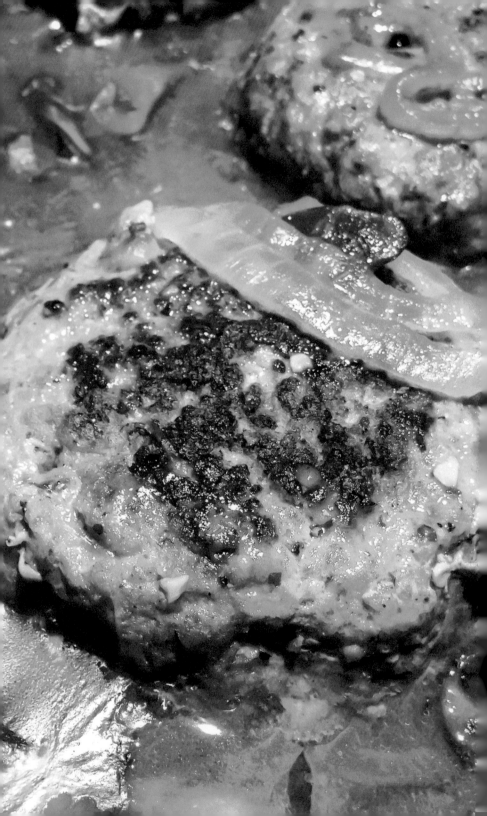

salisbury steak

Servings: 10

2 1/2 lbs lean ground turkey
1 onion, chopped fine
1 cup mushrooms, sliced
3 cloves garlic, minced
3 tbsp extra virgin olive oil
1/4c egg beaters, slightly beaten

2 tbsp Worcestershire sauce
1/4-1/2 cup panko bread crumbs
2 tbsp all-purpose flour
1c low sodium beef stock
1 tbsp parsley
sea salt and pepper

Heat 1 tbsp of extra virgin olive oil in a small skillet over medium-high heat. Add onion and garlic; cook 5 minutes, stirring occasionally. Transfer mixture to a small bowl; cool 5 minutes.

In a large bowl, add ground turkey, panko crumbs, egg, Worcestershire sauce, parsley, salt and pepper, add 1/2 onion & garlic mixture; mix well. Shape into 10 (4oz) oval patties. In same skillet over medium-high heat, add olive oil and brown both sides of the patties. Remove patties from skillet. Set aside.

To make brown gravy or roux: In same skillet with the drippings from turkey burgers, add additional olive oil and heat on medium heat. Add flour to skillet. Stir consistently until flour browns, turning a peanut butter color. You may or may not need to add additional olive oil or butter. Add beef stock or water, mushrooms, onion and garlic mixture. Stir until gravy begins to thicken. Add additional liquid to adjust gravy thickness. Add patties to gravy. Reduce heat to low. Cover and allow patties to simmer for 30 minutes.

Serve with mixed salad, steamed green vegetables and roasted or mashed sweet potatoes. Enjoy!

Nutritional Facts: Nutritional information based on one (1) serving or 1 turkey patty.
Calories: 216 | **Fat:** 18g | **Fiber:** 0g | **Carbs:** 5g | **Protein:** 20g | **Sugar:** 1g

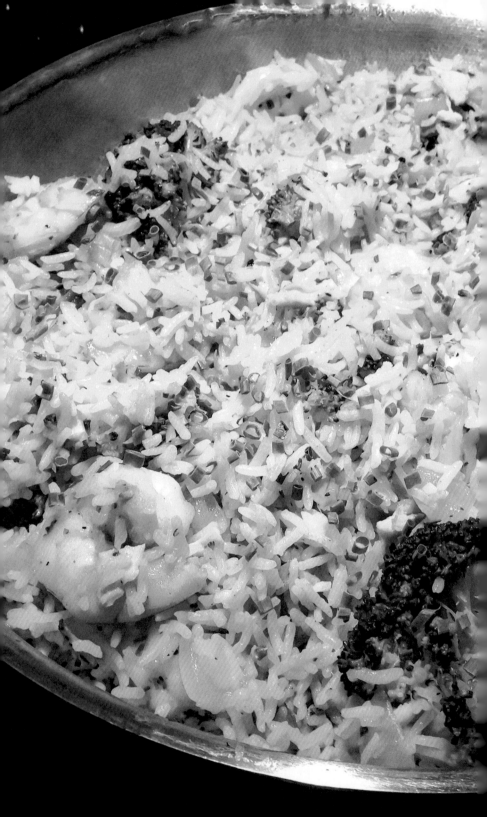

shrimp & broccoli rice

Servings: 8

2-3 cups Jasmine Rice, prepared according to directions.
1 lb large shrimp, peeled & deveined
2-3 cups fresh or steamed fresh frozen broccoli
1/2 cup egg beaters, whisk lightly
2 tbsp extra virgin olive oil
1 medium sweet onion, chopped
2 tbsp green onions or chives
sea salt and black pepper

Make rice the day before. Prepare rice according to directions. Set aside. Add olive oil to large skillet over medium heat. Add onions. Saute for about 3-5 minutes. While sautéing onions, add salt & pepper to egg beaters. Whisk lightly; set aside. Add shrimp to skillet. Saute shrimp until they are almost done. Add fresh or steamed fresh broccoli. Saute for about 5 minutes, stirring constantly.

Push ingredients to one side of the skillet. Add the eggs & quickly scramble eggs. Stir all ingredients together. Add cooked jasmine rice. Stir all ingredients together. Sprinkle with green onions or chives.

Serve with mixed green salad. Enjoy!

Nutritional Facts: Nutritional information based on one (1) serving or 1/2 cup.
Calories: 177 | **Fat:** 4g | **Fiber:** 1g | **Carbs:** 22g | **Protein:** 13g | **Sugar:** 1g

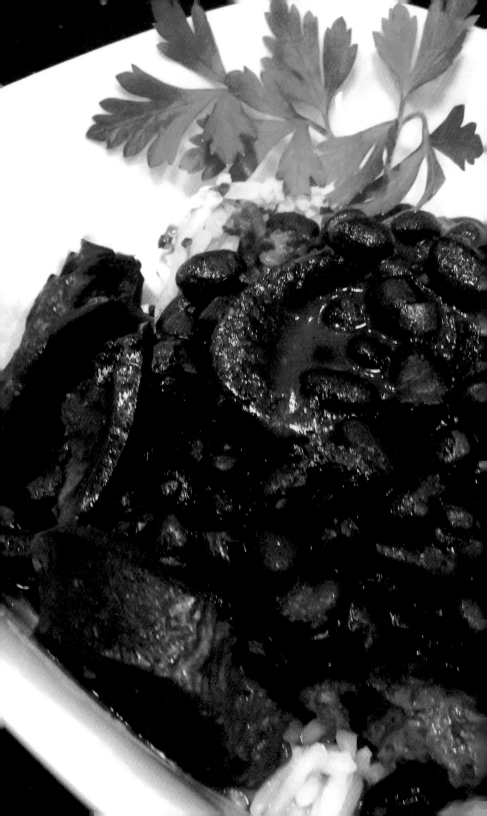

black beans with jasmine rice

Servings: 6-8

1lb black beans (any beans)	chicken stock
1 8oz pkg turkey tasso	4 bay leaves
2 tbsp extra virgin olive oil	1 tsp cayenne pepper
1 large onion, chopped	2 tbsp parsley
1 green bell pepper, chopped	salt and black pepper
4 garlic cloves, chopped	2 cups Jasmine rice
10 cups of water or low sodium	

Rinse beans and pick out all the bad beans. Put beans in large pot. Add 10 cups of water or stock, bay leaves, and put on low heat. In a skillet, heat olive oil over medium heat. Cook tasso or turkey smoke sausage for 5 minutes. Remove from skillet and set aside. Add onions, garlic, and bell pepper to same skillet and saute seasonings for 5 minutes or until slightly translucent. Add cooked seasoning, cayenne pepper, black pepper, salt (to taste) to beans. Stir and cover.

Bring to a boil and then reduce heat to medium-low. Simmer for 2-2 1/2 hours. Add parsley, smoke sausage or turkey tasso and continue to simmer for approximately 30 minutes. *Optional: Try adding cooked/ chopped chicken breast to beans.*

Prepare Jasmine rice according to directions. Serve beans over jasmine rice. Optional: replace jasmine rice with brown rice. Enjoy!

Nutritional Facts: Nutritional information based on one (1) serving or 1/2 cup of beans.
Calories: 347 | **Fat:** 7g | **Fiber:** 16g | **Carbs:** 46g | **Protein:** 24g | **Sugar:** 5g

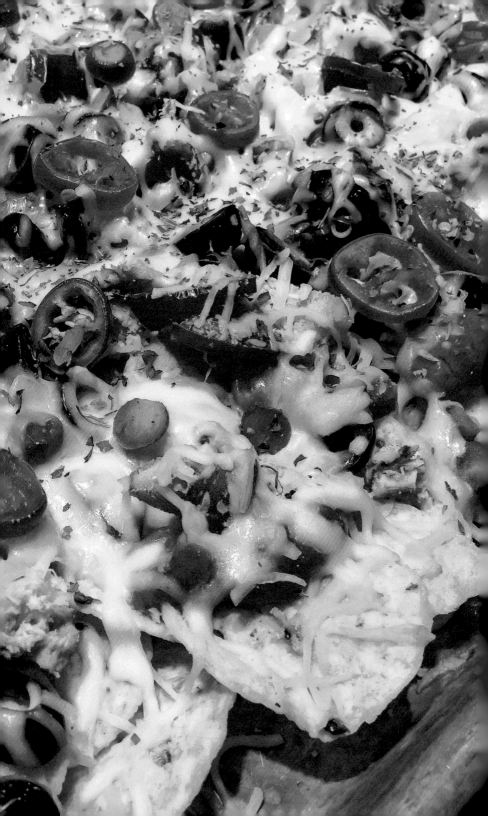

chicken nachos

Servings: 4-6

2 oz (or approx. 48 chips) tostitos bite size corn chips
2 4oz chicken breast, cooked & shredded
1 cup reduced fat sharp cheddar cheese
1 cup reduced fat mozzarella cheese
1 medium tomato, chopped or Fresh Salsa *(recipe on pg. 151)*
1 cup jalapeno peppers
1/2 cup black olives, sliced
1 cup black beans, rinsed & drained or refried beans
low fat sour cream or plain greek yogurt

Preheat oven to 400°F. Arrange the corn chips or chips of choice on a large baking tray. Sprinkle chips with black beans or refried beans, shredded chicken, tomatoes, black olives, cheese, and jalapeño peppers.

Bake nachos for 5-10 minutes or until the cheese is melted. Garnish with sour cream or greek yogurt. As an optional garnish, top with avocado slices. Enjoy!

Nutritional Facts: Nutritional information based on one (1) serving or 12 chips.
Calories: 254 | **Fat:** 13g | **Fiber:** 3g | **Carbs:** 16g | **Protein:** 20g | **Sugar:** 2g

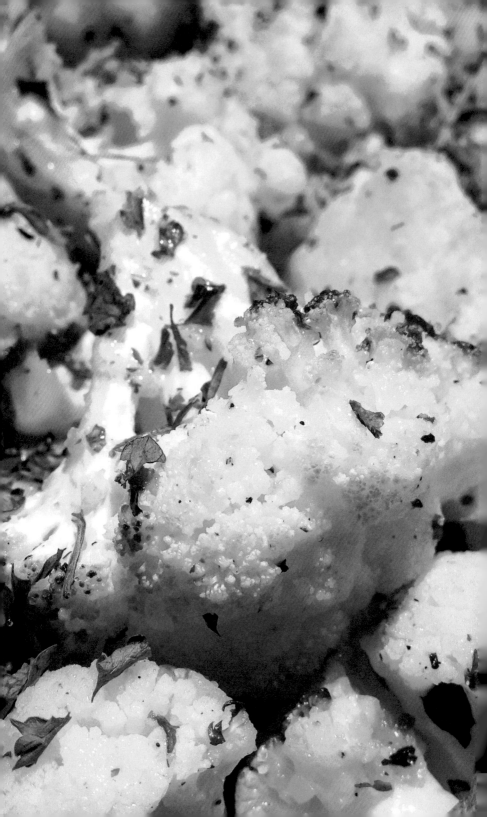

roasted cauliflower

Servings: 8

2 medium head cauliflower, separated into florets
3 garlic cloves, minced
2 tbsp extra virgin olive oil
2 tbsp parsley
1/4-1/2 cup Parmesan cheese, grated
sea salt and black pepper

Preheat oven to 400°F. Spray baking dish with cooking spray. In large mixing bowl, add cauliflower florets, olive oil, garlic, parsley, salt and pepper. Toss well, making sure cauliflower is coated evenly.

Place cauliflower in baking dish and roast for 30-40 minutes. Toss occasionally. Within the final 5-10 minutes of cooking, sprinkle Parmesan cheese and roast cauliflower until tender. Enjoy!

Nutritional Facts: Nutritional information based on one (1) serving or 1/2 cup.
Calories: 88 | **Fat:** 5g | **Fiber:** 4g | **Carbs:** 8g | **Protein:** 5g | **Sugar:** 4g

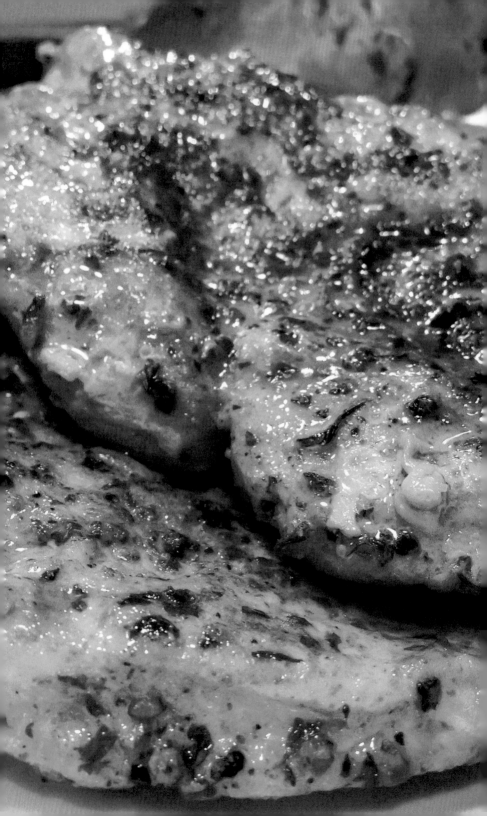

spicy herb chicken breast

Servings: 6

3 5-7oz boneless/skinless chicken breasts, sliced in half (6 breasts)
2-3 tbsp extra virgin olive oil
1 tsp Goya® adobo
2 tsp cayenne pepper
2 tsp black pepper
2 tbsp parsley

In a bowl, mix together the adobo, cayenne pepper, black pepper, and parsley. Season both sides of chicken breasts with seasoning mix and set aside for about 5 minutes. Place seasoned chicken breasts inside ziploc bag. Use meat tenderizer and pound chicken breasts until thin.

In large skillet over medium heat, add olive oil and cook chicken breasts for about 8-10 minutes on each side or until juices run clear.

Enjoy these chicken breasts with steamed vegetables, add to your favorite salads, or make a great sandwich for lunch.

Nutritional Facts: Nutritional information based on one (1) serving or 1 chicken breast.
Calories: 154 | **Fat:** 7g | **Fiber:** 0g | **Carbs:** 1g | **Protein:** 21g | **Sugar:** 0g

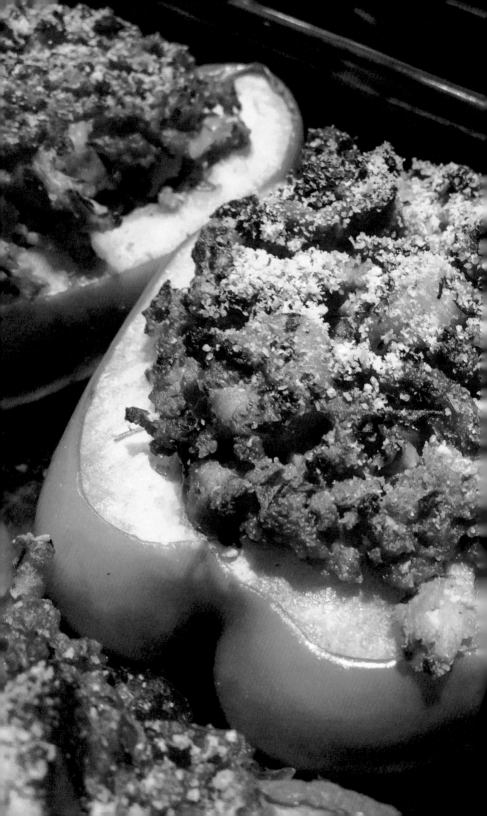

stuffed bell pepper

Servings: 14

7 large green bell peppers, cut in half & seeded
2.5 lbs ground turkey
1 lb crawfish tails
1 8oz package turkey tasso
1 medium sweet onion, chopped
3 garlic cloves, chopped
1 green bell pepper, chopped

2 tbsp extra virgin olive oil
2 tbsp parsley
2 tbsp thyme
1 cup reduced fat cheddar cheese
1 cup panko bread crumbs
1 tsp cayenne pepper
sea salt and pepper

Preheat oven to 350°F. In large skillet over medium heat, add olive oil, onions, garlic, and bell pepper. Saute for 5 minutes. Add ground turkey. Season with salt, black pepper, and cayenne pepper. Cook until ground turkey is cooked. Drain excess water/fat. Add turkey tasso, and cook for 5 minutes. Add peeled/deveined shrimp or crawfish tails, thyme, and parsley. Cook for 2 minutes. Add cheese; stirring in 1/4c at a time. The cheese will help to bind the turkey mixture with the panko crumbs. After cheese is melted and mixed well, add 1/2 cup of panko crumbs. Only add additional panko crumbs depending upon the consistency you want for your stuffing mixture.

Place the bell pepper halves in a baking dish. Stuff each bell pepper half with the turkey stuffing. Lightly sprinkle the top with bread crumbs. Add just a little water to cover the bottom of baking pan. The steam from the water will cook the peppers. Bake for 30-45 minutes. Enjoy!

Nutritional Facts: Nutritional information based on one (1) serving or 1 stuffed pepper.
Calories: 218 | **Fat:** 13g | **Fiber:** 2g | **Carbs:** 10g | **Protein:** 22g | **Sugar:** 3g

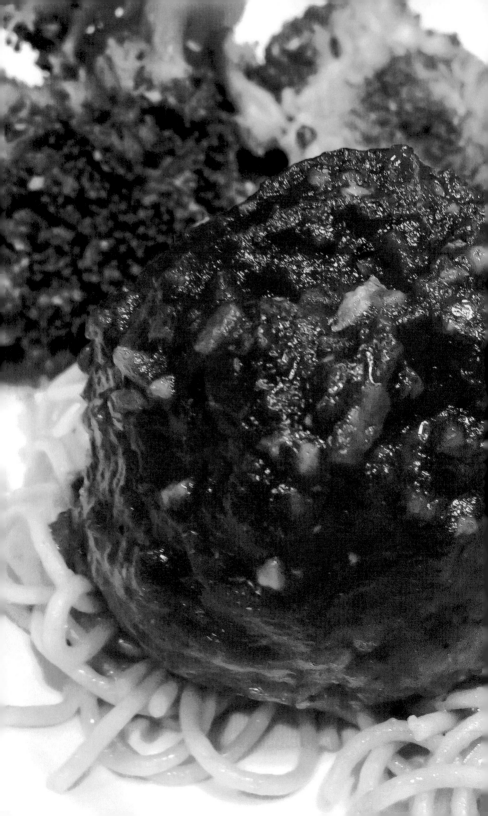

turkey meatballs

Servings: 10

2.5 lbs ground turkey
1 medium sweet onion, chopped
2 garlic cloves, chopped
1 green bell pepper, chopped
2 tbsp extra virgin olive oil
4 tbsp parsley
2 tbsp oregano
2 tbsp thyme
1/4 cup egg beaters or 1 egg

1 cup panko crumbs
1 tsp cayenne pepper
salt and pepper
1 jar of tomato sauce or 2 1/2
cups homemade tomato sauce
1 lb whole wheat angel hair
pasta, prepare according to
directions

Preheat oven to 425°F. In large skillet over medium heat, add 1 tbsp olive oil and 1/2 of chopped onions and garlic. Saute for about 5 minutes. Set aside and let cool.

In large mixing bowl, add ground turkey, saute onions and garlic mixture, egg, 2 tbsp parsley, 1 tbsp oregano, 1 tbsp thyme, panko crumbs, salt and pepper. Mix well and shape into 2.5 oz meatballs. Spray baking sheet or cover baking sheet with foil. Place meatballs on baking sheet. Bake for 30-45 minutes. Remove and set aside.

Tomato Sauce: In large skillet over medium heat, add olive oil and bell pepper. Saute for 5 minutes. Add remaining onion and garlic mixture. Season with salt, black pepper, and cayenne pepper. Add jar tomato sauce or homemade sauce and remaining herbs. Stir well and cook for about 5 minutes. Add meatballs. Cover and simmer sauce for 30-45 minutes. Serve over whole wheat pasta. Enjoy!

Nutritional Facts: Nutritional information based on one (1) serving or 1/2c & 2 meatballs.
Calories: 235 | **Fat:** 17g | **Fiber:** 2g | **Carbs:** 13g | **Protein:** 18g | **Sugar:** 5g

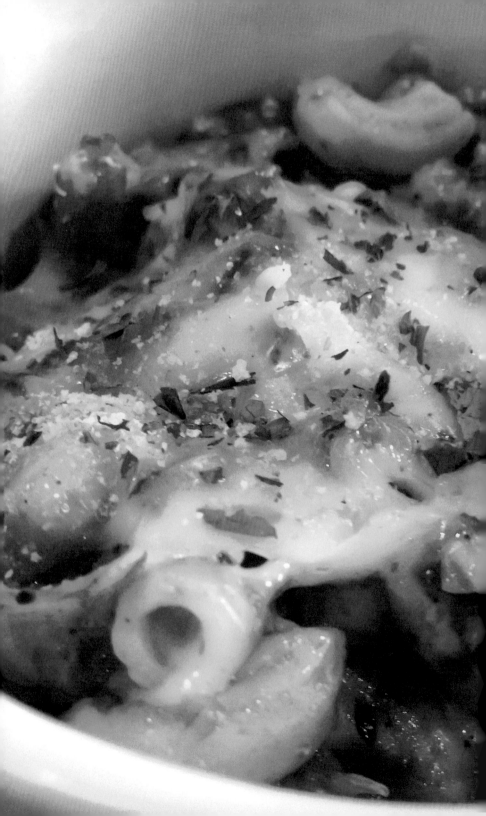

chicken pasta bake

Servings: 8

1 lb whole wheat elbow pasta,
prepare according to directions
1 lb boneless/skinless chicken
breasts, cooked and cubed
1 medium sweet onion, chopped
2 garlic cloves, chopped
1 green bell pepper, chopped
2 tbsp extra virgin olive oil
2 tbsp parsley

2 tsp oregano
2 tsp thyme
2 tsp sweet basil
1 jar of favorite tomato sauce or
homemade tomato sauce
$1^{1/2}$ cup reduced fat colby cheese
1 tsp cayenne pepper
sea salt and pepper

Preheat oven to 350°F. Spray baking dish with cooking spray. Set aside. Cook pasta according to directions. Strain and set aside.

In large skillet over medium heat, season and cook chicken breasts. Remove from skillet. Set aside. Allow chicken breasts to "rest," allowing juices to settle before cutting into cubes.

In same large skillet, add remaining olive oil, onions, garlic, bell pepper, oregano, thyme, and basil. Saute for 5 minutes. Add jar tomato sauce or homemade sauce, cayenne and black pepper. Salt to taste. Stir well and cook for about 5 minutes. Add cubed chicken. Cover and simmer sauce for 30 minutes. Add drained elbow pasta and mix well. Pour half mixture into baking dish and top with 1/2 cup of cheese. Repeat process and top with remaining cheese. Bake for 20-30 minutes or until heated through and cheese has melted.

Sprinkle top with fresh parsley. Enjoy!

Nutritional Facts: Nutritional information based on one (1) serving or 1/4-1/2 cup.
Calories: 208 | **Fat:** 4g | **Fiber:** 10g | **Carbs:** 28g | **Protein:** 14g | **Sugar:** 3g

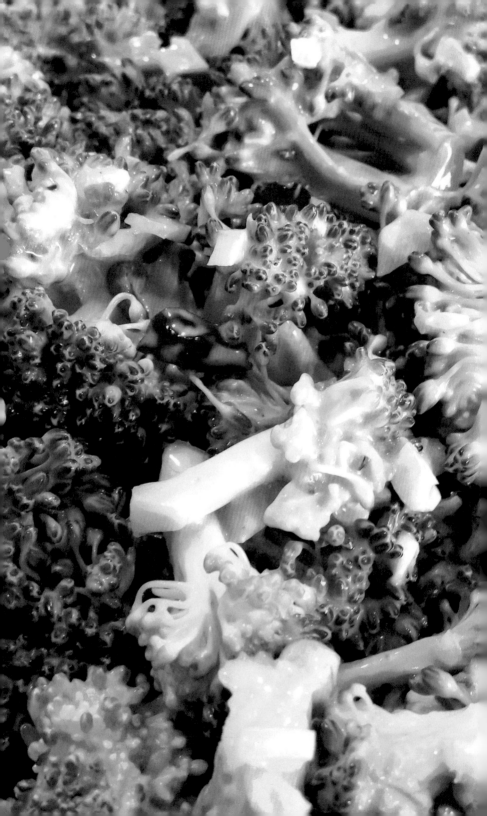

broccoli salad

Servings: 8-10

6 cups broccoli florets
1 medium sweet onion, finely
chopped
1/4 cup craisins
2 tbsp almond slices
6 turkey bacon slices, cooked
and crumbled *(optional)*

Dressing:
1/2 cup light olive oil mayonnaise
1 tbsp olive oil
2 tbsp balsamic vinegar
2 tbsp Splenda® Brown Sugar
black pepper to taste

Separate broccoli florets from broccoli stalks. In large mixing bowl, combine broccoli florets, onions, and craisins. Set aside.

To make dressing: In small bowl, combine all ingredients and mix well. Add dressing in small amounts to broccoli salad (1/4c increments; you should only need to use 1/2c of dressing and can store the remaining for use as homemade salad dressing. The goal is to coat the broccoli well but not oversaturate it with dressing. Add optional turkey bacon crumbles. Mix well. Chill.

When ready to serve, top with almond slices. Enjoy!

Nutritional Facts: Nutritional information based on one (1) serving or 1/2 cup.
Calories: 134 | **Fat:** 7g | **Fiber:** 2g | **Carbs:** 11g | **Protein:** 3g | **Sugar:** 11g

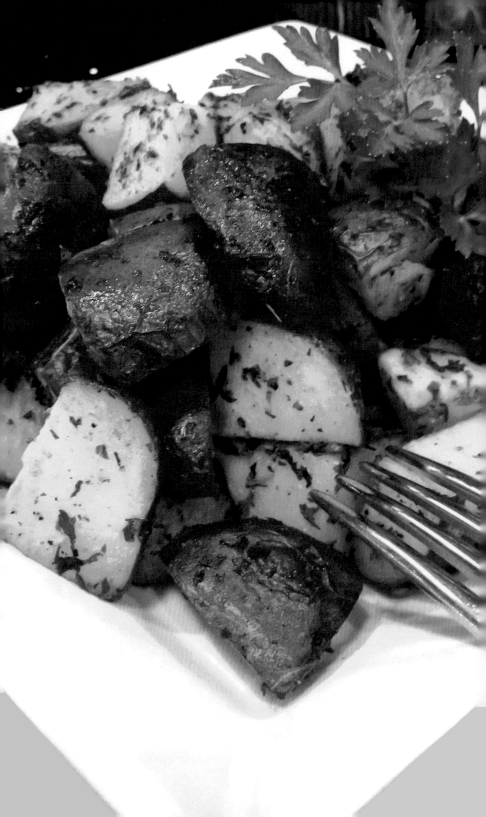

roasted red potatoes

Servings: 8

8 medium red potatoes, cut into 1/2"- 1"thick cubes
2 tablespoon extra virgin olive oil
2 tablespoon parsley
sea salt & black pepper

Preheat oven to 425°F. In large mixing bowl, combine all ingredients and toss. Arrange potato pieces in a single layer on heavyweight rimmed baking sheet or in 13×9-inch baking dish.

Place on middle rack of oven and roast until tender and slightly browned, about 40 minutes.

Nutritional Facts: Nutritional information based on one (1) serving or 1/4-1/2 cup.
Calories: 140 | **Fat:** 4g | **Fiber:** 3g | **Carbs:** 26g | **Protein:** 4g | **Sugar:** 3g

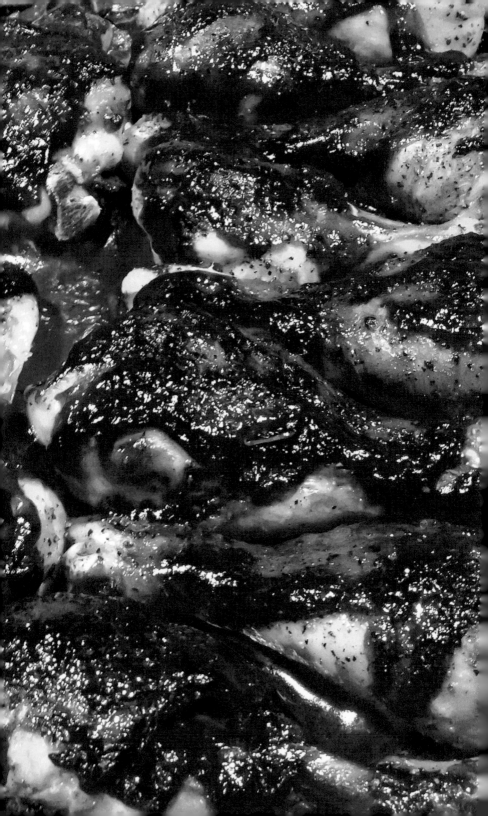

oven baked bbq chicken

Servings: 16

16 chicken drumsticks
2 tbsp extra virgin olive oil
salt and pepper

BBQ Sauce:
1/4 cup ketchup
1/4-1/2 cup Splenda® brown

sugar
2 tbsp balsamic vinegar
2 tbsp water
1 tsp Worcestershire sauce
1/2 tsp paprika
1/2 tsp cayenne pepper
sea salt and black pepper

In small sauce pan, add ketchup, brown sugar, balsamic vinegar, water, Worcestershire sauce, paprika, cayenne pepper, salt, and black pepper. Simmer on low heat until smooth and well blended.

Preheat oven to 425°F. Coat the chicken with olive oil and salt and pepper. Place chicken drumsticks in 13x9 baking dish. Bake for 30-45 minutes. During the last 10 minutes of baking, coat chicken drumsticks with bbq sauce.

Continue baking until a meat thermometer reads 185°F. Enjoy!

Nutritional Facts: Nutritional information based on one (1) serving or 1 drumstick.
Calories: 111 | **Fat:** 6g | **Fiber:** 0g | **Carbs:** 5g | **Protein:** 9g | **Sugar:** 4g

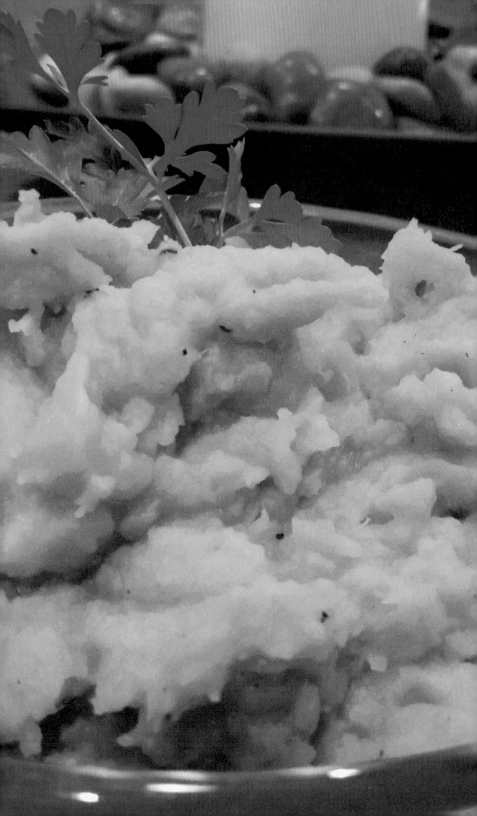

mashed sweet potatoes

Servings: 6-8

6 (4-5lbs) sweet potatoes, peeled and cubed
1 cup unsweetened almond milk
2 tbsp unsalted butter
1 tbsp granulated garlic
1 tbsp parsley
sea salt and black pepper

Add sweet potatoes to large pot. Cover with water. Add salt and bring to a boil. Cook for 20 minutes or until fork tender. Drain.

Return sweet potatoes to large pot. Add butter and 1/4c of almond milk. Begin mashing the sweet potatoes. Slowly add additional almond milk , 1/4 cup at a time until desired texture. Add granulated garlic, salt, black pepper, and parsley. Blend until smooth. Enjoy!

Nutritional Facts: Nutritional information based on one (1) serving or 1/2 cup.
Calories: 95　|　**Fat:** 3g　|　**Fiber:** 2g　|　**Carbs:** 15g　|　**Protein:** 1g　|　**Sugar:** 3g

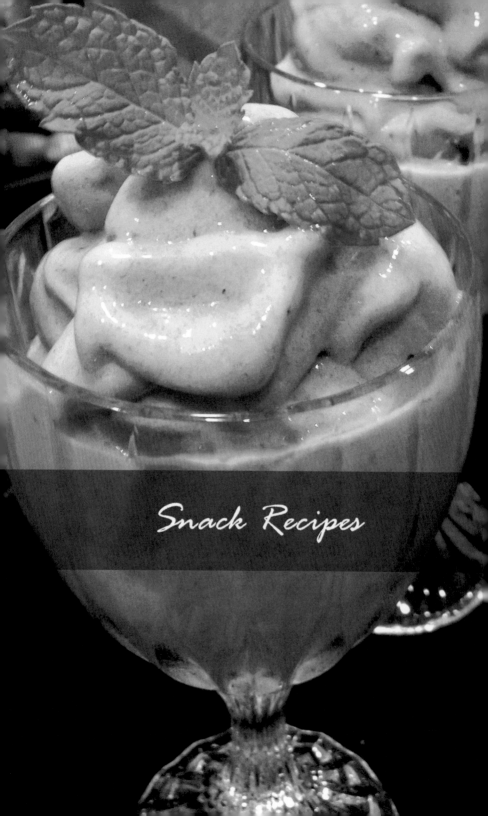

Snack Recipes

snack tip

Snacks are important because they help balance your day. Snacks are little bridges that connect your bodies' fuel to breakfast, lunch, and dinner.

Whether enjoying a great trail mix, fresh fruit, or a smoothie, snacks help you get in the additional nutrients between meals to keep your body properly fueled and your mind focused.

DO NOT SKIP SNACKS!

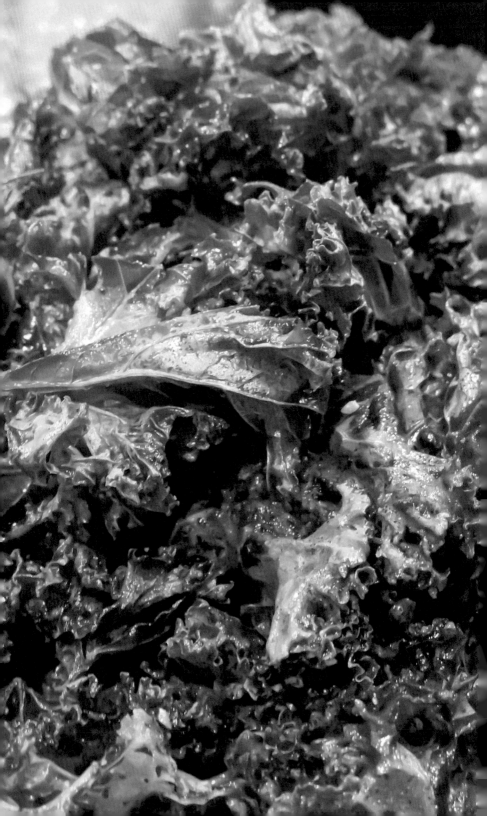

kale chips

Servings: 4-6

8 cups kale, remove leaves from thick stem
1 tbsp extra virgin olive oil
sea salt and black pepper
1 tsp cayenne pepper
Parmesan cheese (optional)

Make sure kale is thoroughly washed and dried before cooking. A salad spinner is ideal to remove all access water from leaves. Remove kale leaves from any remaining hard stems. You want to roast just the kale leaves.

Preheat oven to 250°F. In large mixing bowl, add kale. Drizzle with olive oil. Do a rough mix using your hands or tongs. Sprinkle kale with salt, black pepper, cayenne pepper, or seasonings/herbs of choice. Toss to make sure kale is mixed well. Place kale on baking sheet. Sprinkle with Parmesan cheese. Bake for 15-20 minutes or until edges of kale are light brown or kale is crispy when moved. Enjoy!

Nutritional Facts: Nutritional information based on one (1) serving or 1/2 cup.
Calories: 68 | **Fat:** 5g | **Fiber:** 1g | **Carbs:** 5g | **Protein:** 2g | **Sugar:** 0g

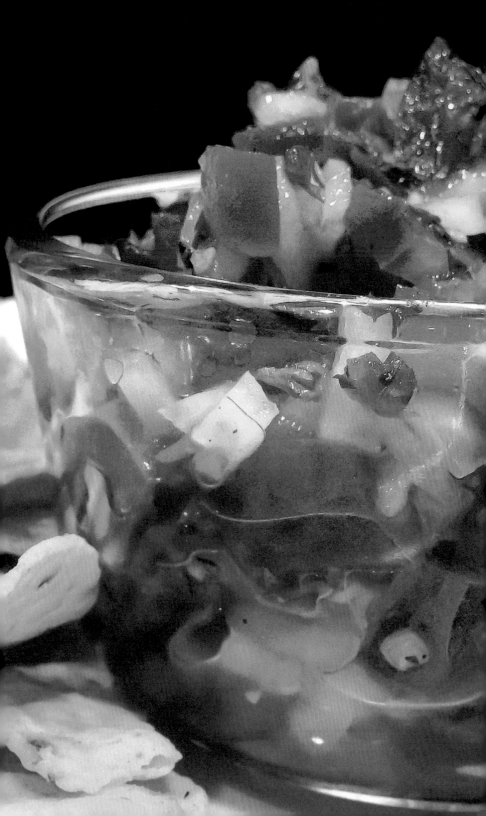

fresh salsa

Servings: 6-8

6 fresh ripe tomatoes, chopped
1 cup sweet onion, chopped
3 cloves of garlic, chopped
1/4-1/2 cup jalapeno peppers, chopped
1/4 cup cilantro
1 tbsp parsley
1 tbsp lime juice
sea salt and black pepper (to taste)

Combine all the ingredients in a large bowl and mix until well blended.
Refrigerate until used. Enjoy!

Nutritional Facts: Nutritional information based on one (1) serving or 1/4-1/2 cup.
Calories: 22 | **Fat:** 0g | **Fiber:** 1g | **Carbs:** 5g | **Protein:** 1g | **Sugar:** 3g

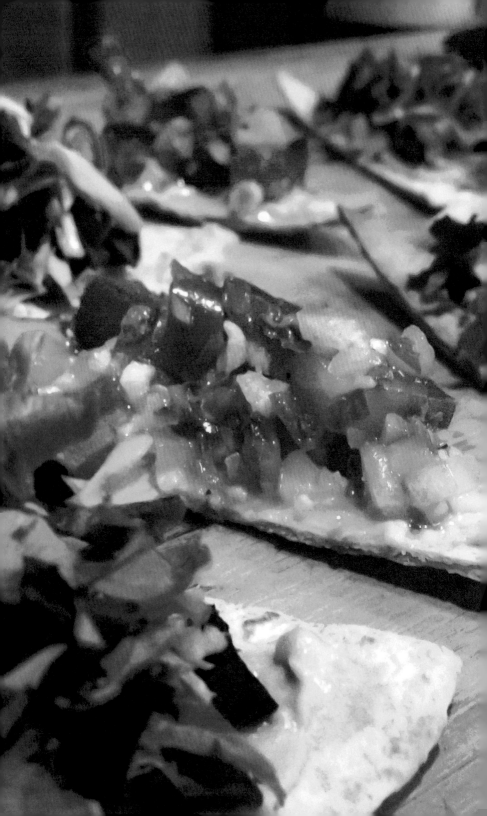

hummus wedges

Servings: 4-6

3 whole wheat tortillas, sliced into 6 wedges per tortilla
3/4 cup Sabra® Roasted Red Pepper Hummus (1 tsp per wedge)
2 cups Spring Mix or Baby Kale & Spinach, chopped
1 cup Fresh Salsa (pg. 151)
2 tbsp Balasamic Vinegar
2 tsp extra virgin olive oil (drizzle over wedges)
sea salt and black pepper

Preheat oven to 375°F. Cut each tortilla into 6 wedges. Place wedges on lightly sprayed cookie sheet. Bake for 8-10 minutes or until lightly brown, just long enough to lightly toast wedges. Remove and allow to cool.

To assemble:
Spread 1/2 tbsp of hummus on each wedge. Drizzle with olive oil. Alternate wedges, topping half with fresh salsa and the other half with spring mix or baby kale/spinach mix. Drizzle balsamic vinegar on top.

Enjoy!

Nutritional Facts: Nutritional information based on one (1) serving or 3-4 wedges.
Calories: 122 | **Fat:** 5g | **Fiber:** 4g | **Carbs:** 17g | **Protein:** 4g | **Sugar:** 3g

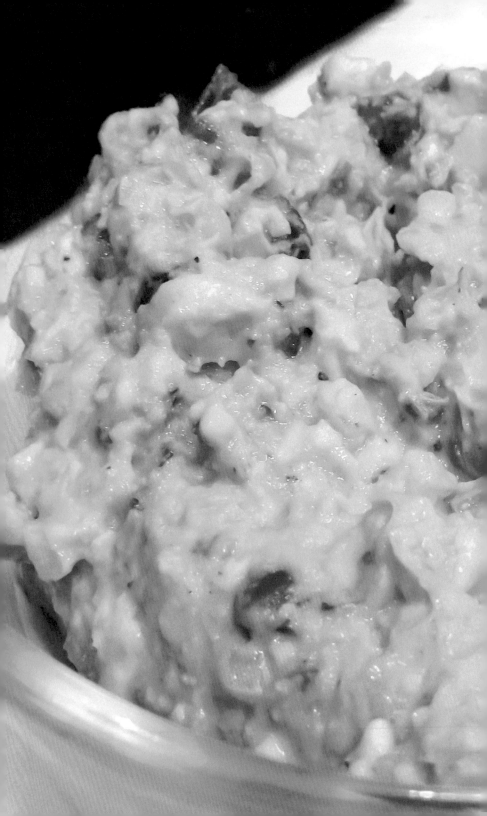

fresh guacamole

Servings: 8

2-3 large rip avocados
1/4-1/2 cup jalapeno peppers, chopped
1/2 small onion, finely chopped
2 cloves of garlic, minced
1 tomato, chopped
2 tbsp cilantro, chopped
1 tbsp fresh lime juice
sea salt and black pepper (to taste)

Cut avocados in half. Remove the seed. Scoop out avocado from peel and put in mixing bowl. Using a fork, roughly mash the avocado. It should be a little chunky. Add the chopped onion, garlic, salt, pepper, lime juice, peppers, and cilantro. Mash/mix a little more.

Cover and refrigerate until ready. Just before serving, add chopped tomatoes to guacamole. Do light mix & serve with tortilla chips, pita chips, or fresh veggies. Enjoy!

Tip: When covering, place plastic wrap directly on top of guacamole to prevent oxidation or air from reaching it & turning it brown.

Nutritional Facts: Nutritional information based on one (1) serving or 1/4 cup.
Calories: 75 | **Fat:** 6g | **Fiber:** 3g | **Carbs:** 7g | **Protein:** 1g | **Sugar:** 0g

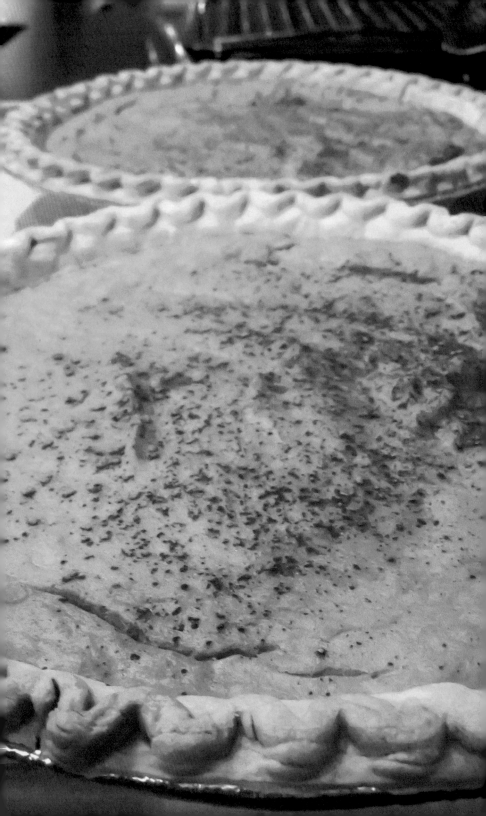

sweet potato pie

Servings: 16

2 - 9" Deep Dish Frozen Pie Crusts
4 medium sweet potatoes, peeled, cubed, and boiled
1/2 cup egg beaters
1 1/4 cups unsweetened almond milk
3/4 cup Splenda®
1/2 tsp salt
1/2 tsp cinnamon
1/2 tsp nutmeg
2 tbsp unsalted butter, melted

Preheat oven to 425°F. Prepare your frozen pie crusts according to the directions. Set aside. Place sweet potatoes in pot and cover with water. Bring to a boil. Boil uncovered until potatoes are fork tender. Drain and set aside to cool. Add sweet potatoes and remaining ingredients in a large bowl and beat until smooth and well blended. Divide the filling in half & pour into both pie crusts.

Bake for 10 minutes, then reduce the heat to 300°F and bake for about 50 minutes more or until the filling is firm.

Nutritional Facts: Nutritional information based on one (1) serving or 1 slice.
Calories: 127 | **Fat:** 6g | **Fiber:** 1g | **Carbs:** 16g | **Protein:** 2g | **Sugar:** 2g

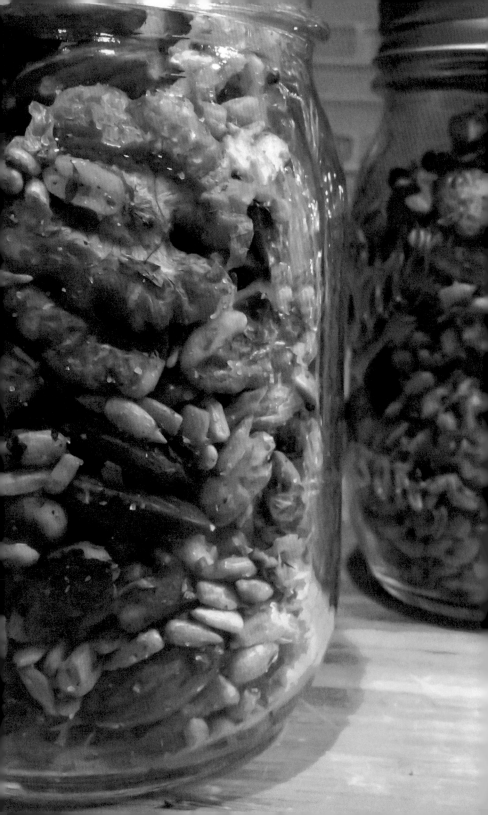

simple trail mix

Servings: 10-12

1 cup Kashi GoLean® Crunch Honey Almond Flax
1/2 cup almonds
1/2 cup walnuts
1/2 cup sunflower seeds
1/2 cup dark chocolate chips
1/4 cup raisins, dried cranberries, or craisins

Combine all the ingredients and store in an airtight container.

Makes approximately 2 1/2 cups - 3 cups.

Nutritional Facts: Nutritional information based on one (1) serving or 1/4 cup.
Calories: 121 | **Fat:** 9g | **Fiber:** 3g | **Carbs:** 10g | **Protein:** 4g | **Sugar:** 4g

Snacks & Treats | **159**

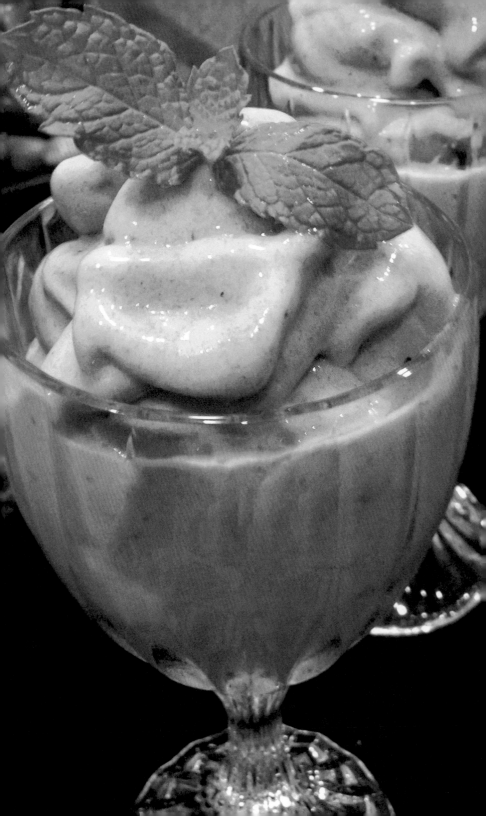

strawberry banana ice cream

Servings: 3

3 medium bananas, cut in 1" pieces, freeze overnight
1 cup frozen strawberries

Blend bananas and strawberries in blender or food processor until the bananas get creamy. You will need to scrape the sides several times, as you blend, to make sure everything mixes well. Depending upon your appliance, you will need to blend on medium-high for several minutes until it the bananas reach a creamy consistency.

Serve immediately or you can place ice cream in a tupperware dish and freeze. We recommend re-blending after freezing when ready to eat.

Be sure to create new favorite ice creams with different fruits, nuts, and even dark chocolate. With the bananas as the base, the possibilities are endless! Enjoy!

Nutritional Facts: Nutritional information based on one (1) serving or 1/2 cup.
Calories: 122 | **Fat:** 1g | **Fiber:** 4g | **Carbs:** 31g | **Protein:** 1g | **Sugar:** 16g

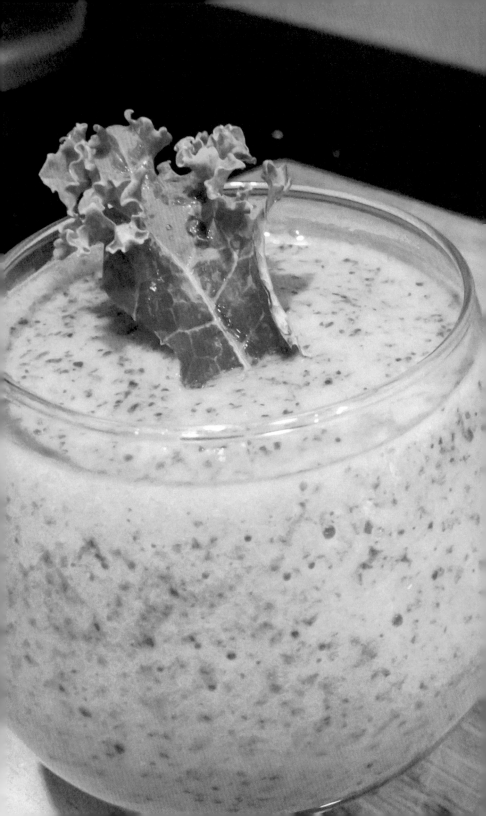

kale & mango smoothie

Servings: 2

1 cup frozen pineapples, strawberries, peaches, and mango fruit
1 medium banana
2 cups kale, chopped
1 cup Almond Milk (vanilla), unsweetened

Place strawberries, banana, kale, and almond milk into a blender. Cover, and puree until smooth. If smoothie is too thick, you can add additional almond milk to reach desired consistency. Enjoy!

Nutritional Facts: Nutritional information based on one (1) serving or 1 cup.
Calories: 126 | **Fat:** 2g | **Fiber:** 4g | **Carbs:** 25g | **Protein:** 2g | **Sugar:** 13g

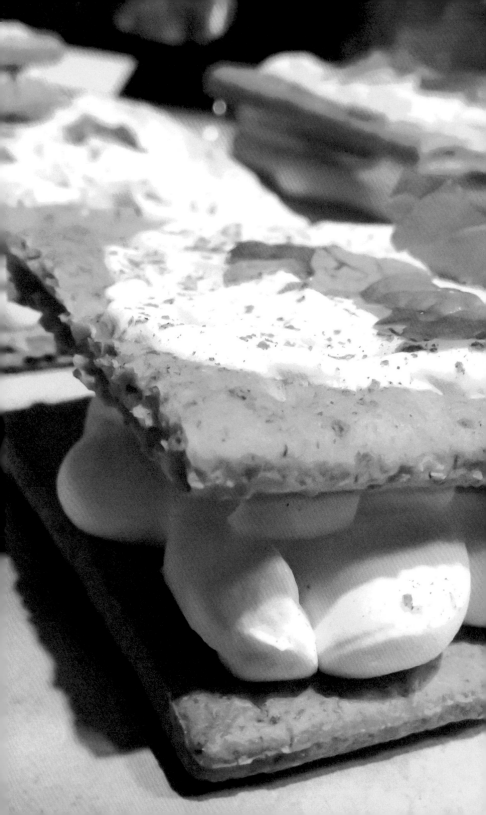

ice cream sandwich

Servings: 8

8 Honey Maid® honey graham crackers, full sheets,
8 tbsp light Cool Whip® or whipped topping
4 fresh mint leaves, chopped
cinnamon for garnish

Break graham cracker in half and place on plate. Spread or pipe
whipped topping on half of the graham cracker. Place another graham
cracker on top, careful not to push it down or smash the sandwich.
Repeat for other full sheet crackers. Add 1 tsp of whipped topping on
top of graham cracker. Spread and sprinkle with cinnamon. Top with
mint leaves. Freeze for 1 hour or until set.

For a real treat, drizzle dark chocolate on top or dip half the sandwich
in dark chocolate. Freeze. Enjoy!

Nutritional Facts: Nutritional information based on one (1) serving or 1 sandwich.
Calories: 78 | **Fat:** 2g | **Fiber:** 1g | **Carbs:** 13g | **Protein:** 1g | **Sugar:** 5g

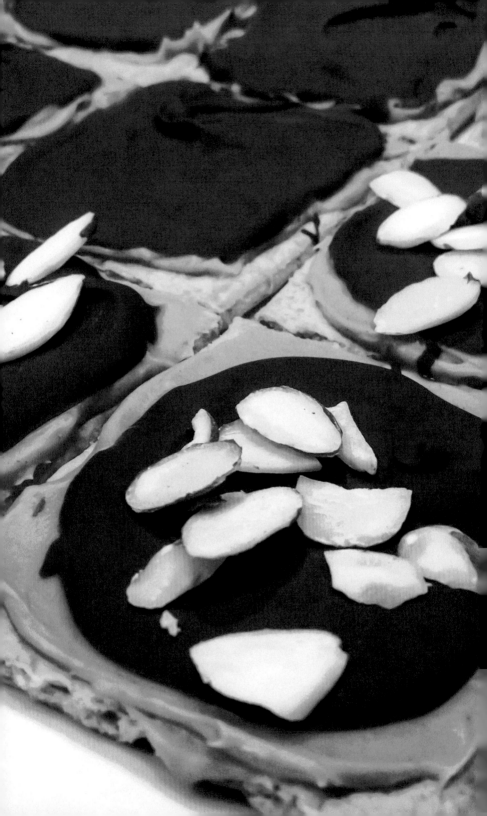

chocolate butter squares

Servings: 12

6 Honey Maid® honey graham crackers, full sheets, divided in halves
4 tbsp peanut butter
2 squares Bakers® Semi Sweet Baking Chocolate squares, melted
almond slices

Break graham cracker in half and spread 1 tsp peanut butter on each graham half sheet. Put in freezer for 5 minutes. Melt chocolate squares according to directions. Remove graham squares from freezer. Drizzle a dime size amount of chocolate on each square. Working quickly and swirl chocolate until it spreads close to edges. Top with almond slices.

Place in freezer to set. Enjoy! Understand, it's HARD to eat just one! Be very aware when you fix these...they are deliciously dangerous!

Nutritional Facts: Nutritional information based on one (1) serving or 1 square.
Calories: 91 | **Fat:** 5g | **Fiber:** 1g | **Carbs:** 10g | **Protein:** 2g | **Sugar:** 5g

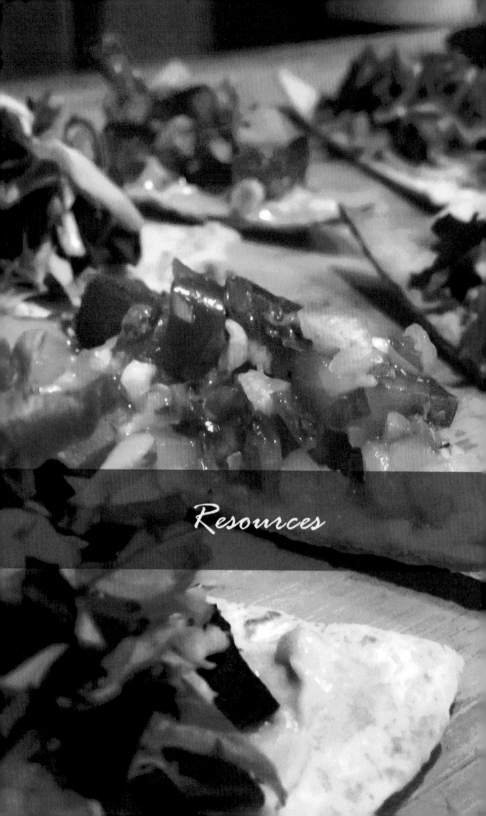

Resources

Bonus

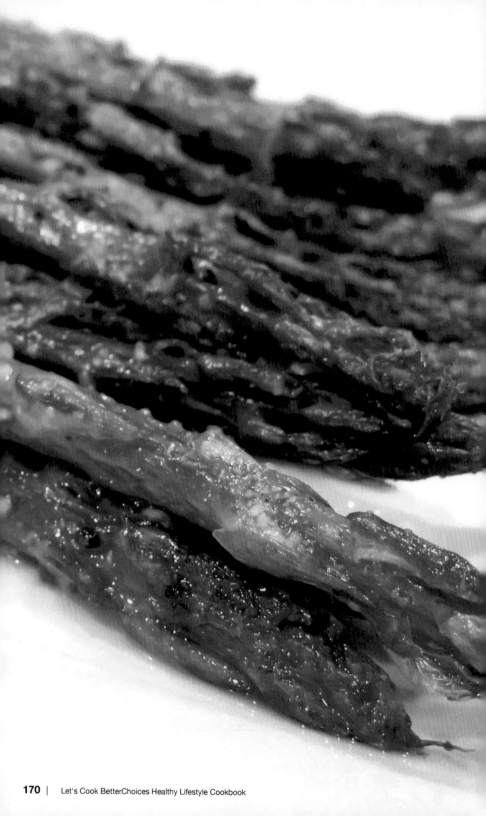

7 day sample menu

Day One:

breakfast:

1c honey nut cheerios
1c unsweetened almond milk
1c or medium piece of fruit
coffee or green tea

snack options:

1c fruit *(1 serving)*
almonds or trail mix
protein shake
+ water

lunch:

turkey sandwich on whole wheat
Sweet Potato or Kale Chips
small green salad
water or unsweetened tea

snack options:

popcorn
fiber one bar
veggies & hummus
+ water

dinner:

roasted chicken
mixed greens
roasted sweet potatoes
water or unsweetened tea

Day Two:

breakfast:

1c steel cut oatmeal
1/2c blueberries or fruit of choice
coffee or green tea

snack options:

1c fruit *(1 serving)*
almonds or trail mix
protein shake
+ water

lunch:

tuna fish salad w/whole wheat pita
Sweet Potato or Kale Chips
small green salad
water or unsweetened tea

snack options:

popcorn
fiber one bar
veggies & hummus
+ water

dinner:

turkey meatloaf
2c green salad
sautéed asparagus
water or unsweetened tea

Day Three:

breakfast:

1 egg + 1/4c Egg Beaters
2 whole wheat bread slices
2 tomato & avocado slices
coffee or green tea

snack options:

1c fruit *(1 serving)*
almonds or trail mix
protein shake
+ water

lunch:

grilled chicken salad
balsamic vinaigrette dressing
water or unsweetened tea

snack options:

popcorn
fiber one bar
veggies & hummus
+ water

dinner:

1c red beans
1/4c jasmine rice
2c mixed green salad
water or unsweetened tea

Day Four:

breakfast:

2 whole grain waffles
1 tbsp natural peanut butter
1c or medium piece of fruit
coffee or green tea

snack options:

1c fruit *(1 serving)*
almonds or trail mix
protein shake
+ water

lunch:

turkey sandwich on whole wheat
sweet potato or kale chips
small green salad
water or unsweetened tea

snack options:

popcorn
fiber one bar
veggies & hummus
+ water

dinner:

grilled tilapia w/sautéed peppers
corn succotash
2c mixed green salad
water or unsweetened tea

Day Five:

breakfast:

1c honey nut cheerios
1c unsweetened almond milk
1c or medium piece of fruit
coffee or green tea

snack options:

1c fruit *(1 serving)*
almonds or trail mix
protein shake
+ water

lunch:

grilled chicken salad
balsamic vinaigrette dressing
water or unsweetened tea

snack options:

popcorn
fiber one bar
veggies & hummus
+ water

dinner:

4oz baked chicken Parmesan
1c glazed carrots
1c roasted cauliflower
water or unsweetened tea

Day Six:

breakfast:

6oz plain greek yogurt
1/2c Kashi Go Lean Cereal or granola
1/c fruit of choice
coffee or green tea

snack options:

1c fruit *(1 serving)*
almonds or trail mix
protein shake
+ water

lunch:

tuna fish salad w/whole wheat pita
Sweet Potato or Kale Chips
small green salad
water or unsweetened tea

snack options:

popcorn
fiber one bar
veggies & hummus
+ water

dinner:

sautéed tilapia & vegetable pizza
2c mixed green salad
water or unsweetened tea

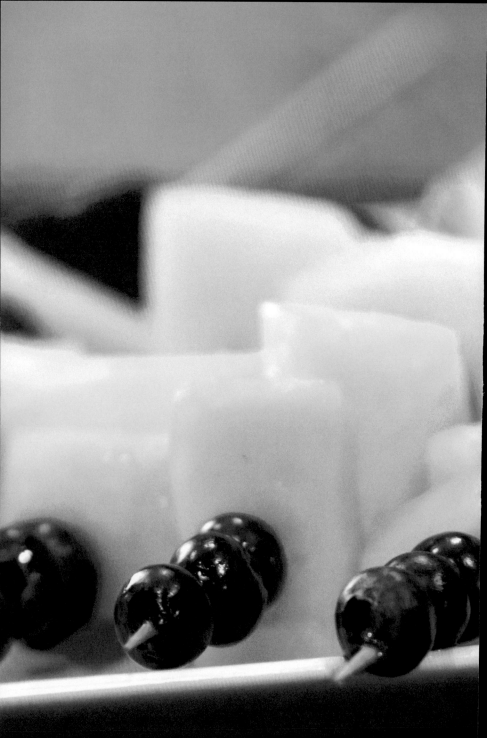

Day Seven:

breakfast:

1 egg + 1/4c Egg Beaters
2 slices turkey bacon (baked)
2 tomato & avocado slices
2 slices whole wheat english muffins
coffee or green tea

snack options:

1c fruit *(1 serving)*
almonds or trail mix
protein shake
+ water

lunch:

peanut butter & jelly sandwich
sweet potato or kale chips
water or unsweetened tea

snack options:

popcorn
fiber one bar
veggies & hummus
+ water

dinner:

fish taco salad w/whole wheat tortilla
1c black beans
fresh salsa
water or unsweetened tea

5 tips to create your weekly menu plan:

1. Add healthy protein sources.
Plan on fish twice a week. Include beans weekly. Why? Because beans are superior sources of both protein & fiber.

2. Veggies! Veggies! Fruit.
Adding vegetables & fruit to each meal will ensure you get your proper nutrients, including essential vitamins. Vegetables & fruit help to keep you full. Whether for main meals or snacks, vegetables and fruit are a MUST!

3. Add whole grain sources.
It's not about cutting carbs but getting the right sources of carbs. Whole grain options include whole grain pastas, breads, oatmeal, cereals, and more.

4. Limit sugary drinks.
Water is perfect for every meal! We highly recommend it. Other good choices include low fat milk, unsweetened teas or lemonade, & vegetable juices.

5. Try one new recipe a week.
Put your new knowledge to work & create your own healthier favorites!

Dairy
(2-3 SERVINGS)

Fats / Oils
SPARINGLY

Protein
(2-3 SERVINGS)

Vegetables
(3-5 SERVINGS)

Whole Grains
(6-11 SERVINGS)

Fruit
(2-4 SERVINGS)

what's on your plate?

That is usually the second or third question we are asked after sharing our weight loss story. What did you eat? What did you have to give up? Most people are pleasantly surprised when we say we still eat the foods we love! Truth is, we didn't give up anything!

Let us explain.

Life is about balance. Life is about experience. It is in the balance and experience of life, that you create your lifestyle. It's important to have balance in your nutritional health and have the experience of indulging or treating yourself to old & new food experiences.

In our approach to BetterChoices, we knew enjoying food was going to be key to our healthier lifestyle success. We realized this change did not mean we could not enjoy "indulgences," it just meant we had to enjoy them in moderation.

What do we mean by "moderation?" Glad you asked! We've included a healthy plate diagram based on the USDA's Center for Nutrition Policy and Promotion dietary recommendations. It's important to fuel your body with healthier sources and proper servings of

protein, vegetables, fruit, whole grains, dairy, and healthy fats. Each group provides your body with essential nutrients that keep your body properly fueled and operating. Whether losing weight or creating a healthier lifestyle, dietary balance is key to your overall health & wellness.

The healthy food plate diagram illustrates the five main food groups to guide you in creating a dietary balance. Each food group includes the daily serving recommendations. You will notice on the next page, we've included some of the most popular items in each food group.

Based on the foods YOU love, create your very own weekly meal plan and make BetterChoices when selecting ingredients, as well as, preparing and consuming the proper servings. Slight reductions or increases can be made based on your daily caloric intake requirement relevant to your height, weight, activity level, and weight loss goals.

We encourage you to consult your physician regarding your personal dietary recommendations.

Visit **www.choosemyplate.gov** for additional resources.

vegetables

- artichokes
- arugula
- asparagus
- bean sprouts
- beets
- bell peppers
- black beans
- blackeye peas
- bok choy
- broccoli
- brussels sprouts
- cabbage
- carrots
- cauliflower
- celery
- collard greens
- corn
- cucumber
- eggplant
- fennel
- garbanzo beans
- garlic
- great northern beans
- green leaf lettuce
- iceberg lettuce
- kale
- kidney beans
- lima beans
- leeks
- lentil
- mushrooms
- mustard greens
- navy beans
- okra
- onions
- parsnips
- peas
- pinto beans
- potatoes
- pumpkin
- radishes
- red leaf cabbage
- red leaf lettuce
- red peppers
- romaine lettuce
- spinach
- squash
- sweet potatoes
- tomatoes
- turnips
- zucchini

fruit

- apple
- apricots
- avocado
- bananas
- blackberries
- blueberries
- cantaloupe
- cherries
- coconut
- cranberries
- dates
- figs
- grapefruit
- grapes
- honeydew melon
- kiwi
- lemons
- limes
- mangos
- nectarines
- oranges
- papayas
- passion fruit
- peaches
- pears
- pineapple
- plums
- pomegranate
- raspberries
- strawberries
- watermelon

fats & oils

- canola oil
- corn oil
- olive oil
- safflower oil
- soybean oil
- sunflower oil
- coconut oil
- peanut oil
- butter

protein

- lean beef, pork, lamb, veal
- ground beef, pork lamb
- chicken
- tofu
- turkey
- ground chicken
- ground turkey
- veggie burgers

- catfish
- clams
- cod
- crab
- crawfish
- flounder
- halibut
- lobster
- mackerel
- mahi mahi
- oyster
- perch
- salmon
- sardines
- scallops
- sea bass
- shrimp
- snapper
- swordfish
- tilapia
- trout
- tuna

- almonds
- cashews
- hazelnuts
- mixed nuts
- peanuts
- peanut butter
- pecans
- pistachios
- pumpkin seeds
- sesame seeds
- sunflower seeds
- walnuts

whole grains

- amaranth
- brown rice
- buckwheat
- bulgur
- cornbread
- corn tortillas
- couscous
- millet
- oatmeal
- popcorn
- whole grain cereal
- muesli
- rolled oats
- quinoa
- sorghum
- triticale
- whole-grain barley
- whole grain cornmeal
- whole corn tortillas
- whole rye
- whole wheat/whole grain bread, pita, sandwich buns, & rolls
- whole grain crackers
- whole wheat pasta
- whole grain noodles
- whole grain tortillas
- wild rice

dairy

- 1% or skim milk
- almond milk
- soy/rice milk
- low/fat-free yogurt
- cottage cheese
- ricotta cheese
- eggs
- egg whites
- sour cream
- cream cheese
- reduced fat cheese

acknowledgements

Through Him, ALL things are possible. With Him, ALL things are blessed. In Him, all things live in abundance, full of grace and filled with divine love.

We are so thankful to God. We are blessed to have this opportunity to serve and share ourselves and our life with you. Our journey has been filled with so many twists and turns, ups and downs, tests and testimonies, that when we look back, we are amazed at how far we've come! We know it is only by God's grace and His mercy, that we live and are able to share our passion of teaching, motivating, and inspiring others to live a healthier life.

We thank God for each other. Every day is truly a new adventure filled with love and laughter. To say we are together ALL DAY, EVERY DAY (no joking...24 hours a day, 7 days a week, 52 weeks a year, leap year, bathroom breaks, etc...we are tighter than panty hose too small! lol!), it is never a moment where we would prefer to be anywhere else. These 18 years have been absolutely amazing! We have cooked a lot and have eaten even more! Whether at our heaviest or our healthiest, we have been each others' support and motivation! There is absolutely nothing we can't do!

To Our Parents Cynthia, Gladys, Buddy, & Mary: Thank you for loving us so much and teaching us how to spread our wings and fly. For both of us, God blessed us with parents who taught us both the meaning of hard work and the importance of living a life of integrity & respect. We grew up knowing NOTHING was impossible...maybe a singing career, but everything else under the horizon was available to us!

You taught us to believe in our dreams, work hard, and always serve ourselves and others with grace, dignity, and genuine care. You said laughter was the key to the soul and to never take ourselves too seriously, that we forget to laugh. We love you. Thank you.

To Our Boys, Eric & Chris: We love you so much! God truly blessed us when He gave us you. The gift of your lives inspires us to be the best we can be. You have always been our inspiration and motivation to live a healthier and more active life. You make us proud when we see you reading nutritional labels, measuring your serving sizes, and making your own betterchoices.

We thank you for your sacrifice and willingness to share our time with you so we could be there for someone else. We love you very much. You are the center of our joy.

To Our Brother, Marcel and Sisters, Zalema & Jacqueline: What can we say but Thank You! Y'all have been with us on this journey from the very beginning! Whether we were all rolling out to an all-you-can-eat-buffet or becoming BetterChoices taste testers, we truly appreciate all your love and support. We love y'all for always being willing to try something new when you come over for dinner. We are so grateful to have you in our lives. Your support and encouragement means the world to us. We love you!

To my Dad, Marcel Sr.: Thank you for loving me unconditionally. You taught me, no matter the circumstance, never give up. I love you.

To Our Extended Family, All of Our Friends & Supporters: Y'all are the best! So many of you have been our friends since kindergarten! Lord knows, that was a long, long, looooong time ago! Kevin, Roger, Rachel, Archie, Mike - our road dawgs! So many adventures! So many foodcations! So much fun!

From day one, each of you made us feel so special and so loved. You never judged us. You always made time for us - whether celebrating our joys or being with us in our pains, you have always been there. We love you and cherish you. Thank you for all of your support, encouragement, restaurant recommendations, and most of all, your honesty and love. Thank you! Thank you! Thank you!

To the nurses who laughed at me: I want to thank you from the bottom of my heart. Who knows where I would be had you not made a spectacle of my weight. Your laughter was the catalyst I needed to wake me up! For so long, we lived our lives not caring about the foods we ate or the lack of activity in our lives.

In that moment, I was angry. I was also grateful. That was the defining moment I needed to motivate us to change our lives. Thank you.

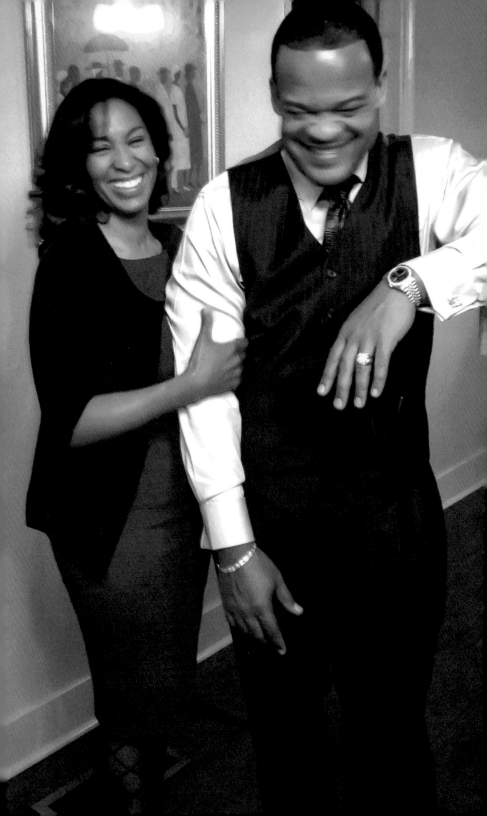

about the authors

ERIC J. BEAL, SR., is the co-founder of BetterChoices, LLC. Eric is a motivational speaker, healthy lifestyle coach & expert, author, and entrepreneur. His inspirational weight loss journey began in 2006, when during a doctor's visit, he was shocked to discover his weight had ballooned to 400 pounds. Determined to gain control of his life, Eric immediately embarked on a systematic process that led to a 150-pound weight loss.

A New Orleans native, Eric proudly served five years with the United States Army. He is an honored Gulf War combat veteran and recipient of the Kuwaiti Liberation Medal. With over 20 years experience in asset recovery, Eric owned & operated Professional Asset Recovery, a commercial collection agency. Most importantly, Eric is a devoted husband and father. "My weight loss success is about weight and so much more. It is about transforming & improving the quality of my life."

MALEKA J. BEAL, is the co-founder of BetterChoices, LLC. Maleka is a motivational speaker, healthy lifestyle coach & expert, author, and entrepreneur. Maleka, whose own weight topped 276 pounds, put aside all her excuses and made the CHOICE to join Eric, resulting in her own incredible weight loss of 138 pounds.

Also a native of New Orleans, Maleka owns and operates a small, branding/graphic design studio, MJB Design studio. Her greatest joy and lifetime blessing is that of being a wife and mother. As a couple, Eric and Maleka bring a unique perspective and approach to life coaching, healthy living & wellness, weight loss, relationship, communicating, parenting, and so much more.

"We are on a mission! BetterChoices provides an opportunity for us to teach and inspire others to change their lives one betterchoice at a time." Eric and Maleka's success story has been featured or shared in Essence Magazine, CNN's HLN, The Dr. Oz Show, The Oprah Show, local newspaper publication and they have appeared on local television, radio, and online blogs, blog radio and podcasts.

For more information about BetterChoices or on their healthy lifestyle coaching and programs, visit **www.betterchoices.co**.

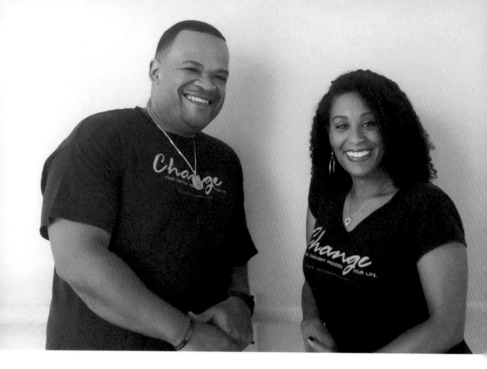
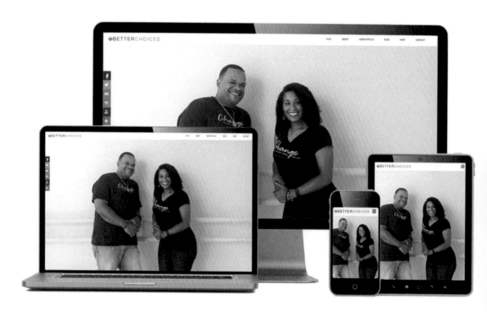

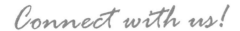
Connect with us!

WHAT IS BETTERCHOICES?

Glad you asked. It's a LIFESTYLE.

BetterChoices is not a diet. It's not a pill, shake, or exercise/product gimmick. It is not a quick fix. Nor, is it a "weight loss" program.

At it's core, BetterChoices is about improving your health and overall wellness. It's about raising your awareness and identifying the lifestyle factors that are currently affecting your health, wellness, & weight loss struggles. We call these tipping points. Tipping points, by logical definition, are small things that make a big difference. We help you identify your specific tipping points. Once identified, we educate you on what they are, how you can change them, and why you should change them. As a result, you experience a "shift" in your mindset and weight loss becomes a tremendous side effect.

WHAT WE DO

BetterChoices is a healthy lifestyle coaching program and online community focused on teaching, motivating, & empowering individuals to live healthier through the process of making BetterChoices. We provide healthy lifestyle individual & group coaching, motivational speaking, healthy lifestyle cookbooks, tips, recipes, and additional resources through our healthy lifestyle blogs.

OUR MISSION

Our goal is simple — to help you obtain optimal health. We want to show you how you can create a healthier lifestyle that will help you improve and control your blood pressure, glucose, and cholesterol. Truth is, you CAN improve your health. Our goal is to educate & empower you to do it.

To get started or to find out more information about our coaching programs, benefits, and more, please visit us **www.betterchoices.co**.

Facebook/Twitter/Instagram/YouTube: @betterchoicesco

resources

FDA **"Food. How to Understand and Use the Nutritional Facts Label."** U.S. Food and Drug Administration, n.d. Web Mar. 2013 <http://www.livestrong.com/article/536193-how-to-lower-your-sugar-intake-to-lose-weight/>

USDA **"What Foods Are in the Fruit Group?"** *What are Fruit?*, ChooseMyPlate.gov, n.d. Web Mar. 21, 2013 <http://www.choosemyplate.gov/food-groups/fruits.html>

CDC **"Healthy Eating for a Healthy Weight"** *Centers for Disease control and Prevention*, Centers for Disease Control and Prevention, 25 Oct. 2012 Web Mar. 21, 2013 <http://www.cdc.gov/healthyweight/healthy_eating/index.html>

"Why Breakfast Is the Most Important Meal of the Day" *WebMD*. WebMD, n.d. Web Jan. 0000 to Mar. 2013 <http://www.webmd.com/food-recipes/most-important-meal>

"Cooking Oils" *Whole Foods Market*. Whole Foods Market, n.d. Web Jan. Mar. 21, 2013 <http://www.webmd.com/food-recipes/most-important-meal>

"Cooking Fats and Oil Types, Smoking Points of FAts and Oils, Monunsaturated Fats, Polyunsaturated Fats, Trans Fatty Acids" *Web Log Post.* Cooking Fats and Oil Types, Smoking Points o Fats and Oils, Monunsaturated Fats, Polyunsaturated Fats, Trans Fatty Acids, n.d. Web Jan. Mar. 21, 2013 <http://whatscookingamerica.net/Information/CookingOilTypes.htm>

Soenarie, Angelique **"Guide to 8 Healthy Oils for Cooking"** *AzCentral.com*. Azcentral.com, 19 Oct. 2011. Web Mar. 21, 2013 <http://www.azcentral.com/style/hfe/food/articles/2011/10/19/20111019guide-healthy-oils-cooking.html?nclick_check=1>

Rose, Gianna **"How to Lower Your Sugar Intake to Lose Weight"** *Web Blog Post. Livestrong.com.* Livestrong.com, 5 Sept. 2011. Web Mar. 21, 2013 <http://www.azcentral.com/style/hfe/food/articles/2011/10/19/20111019guide-healthy-oils-cooking.html?nclick_check=1>

Thank You!

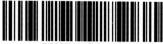

Made in the USA
Middletown, DE
13 December 2016